Comprehensive Manuals in Radiology

Harold G. Jacobson, editor

W. J. Weston · D. G. Palmer

Soft Tissues
of the Extremities

A Radiologic Study
of Rheumatic Disease

with 171 figures

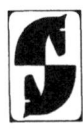

Springer-Verlag
New York Heidelberg Berlin

SERIES EDITOR

Harold G. Jacobson, M.D. Professor and Chairman, Department of Radiology, Montefiore Hospital Medical Center, Bronx, New York 10467

AUTHORS

W. J. Weston, M.B., Ch.B., F.R.C.P. (Edin.), F.R.C.R.A., D.M.R.D. Visiting
Radiologist, Hutt Hospital, Lower Hutt, New Zealand, Member of the International Skeletal Society
D. G. Palmer, M.D., M.R.C.P., F.R.A.C.P., Associate Professor in Medicine,
and Physician in Charge, Rheumatic Diseases Unit, Department of Medicine, University of Otago Medical School, Dunedin, New Zealand

Library of Congress Cataloging in Publication Data

Weston, Windsor John.
    Soft tissues of the extremities.

    (Comprehensive manuals in radiology)
    Includes bibliographical references and index.
    1. Rheumatoid arthritis—Diagnosis. 2. Joints—Radiography.
I. Palmer, David G., joint author. II. Title. III. Series. [DNLM:
1. Extremities—Anatomy and histology. 2. Extremities—Radiography.
3. Rheumatism—Radiography. WE800 W536s]
RC933.W5   616.7′2′0757   77-7951

Softcover reprint of the hardcover 1st edition 1978

9 8 7 6 5 4 3 2 1

ISBN-13: 978-1-4612-6253-4   e-ISBN-13: 978-1-4612-6251-0
DOI: 10.1007/978-1-4612-6251-0

This is dedicated to

Professor W. P. Gowland
Professor W. E. Adams
Dr. O. C. Moller

Mirdza Palmer
and
Elizabeth Weston

Foreword

During the past decade there has been a burgeoning of interest in arthritis and related rheumatic diseases. The speciality of rheumatology, once regarded as a "Cinderella" speciality, is now one of the leading specialties in internal medicine. Indeed, just as infant mortality is a good index of the general health of a community, so a University Medical School can be similarly judged by the quality of its Department of Rheumatology. Perhaps no other specialty has helped to advance knowledge in medicine as has rheumatology

One might have thought that little could be added to the clinical and radiologic description of one of the most studied diseases in rheumatology—rheumatoid arthritis. There are several excellent large radiology textbooks on bones and joints, and it is surprising that yet another book has been published. However, the reader will soon appreciate on reading this superb radiologic text on rheumatoid arthritis that here is something new and quite different from what has been published in the past. The combination of clinician and radiologist has produced a textbook which will become a standard reference on the subject. The authors are both well known in their respective fields and they have concentrated on the early changes in the disease—not only those in the articular surfaces but also those in the soft tissues. In 1948 the late Dr Philip Ellman coined the term "rheumatoid disease," to indicate the systemic nature of rheumatoid arthritis. It is my belief that Professor David Palmer and Dr John Weston have created another important new concept of 'extra-capsular' rheumatoid arthritis, drawing attention to the clinical and radiologic importance of structures surrounding the joints.

The book is not only well written, and well illustrated, but also contains a singularly up-to-date bibliography. At present it is fashionable to decry the teaching of regional anatomy, but Deans of Medical Schools who are poised ready to limit the number of hours devoted to this undergraduate subject would be well advised to read this book before doing so. The authors also make useful reference to other than standard radiologic procedures and, in so doing, bring alive what to many is a somewhat dull and mudane diagnostic procedure.

Congratulations to the authors are superfluous: their book does this for them.

Glasgow, Scotland   W. WATSON BUCHANAN

Preface

Interest in the radiologic aspects of rheumatoid arthritis has been stimulated over the last three decades by descriptions of the changes which may occur at the articular surfaces of the involved joints. Such descriptions have led to earlier diagnosis, better differentiation of rheumatoid arthritis from related arthritic disorders, standardization of the stage of disease, objective assessment of progression, and a better understanding of the pattern of the disease process itself (4, 5, 21). Texts such as those by Forrester and Nesson (8) and Berens and Lin (3) have covered the broad field of radiologic diagnosis, in joint disease. There is, nevertheless, room for improvement in radiologic diagnosis, for it is the involvement of the soft tissues, not the articular erosions, which is the first radiologic change to result from joint inflammation (6). The contribution that the more detailed radiologic study of the soft tissues can make to earlier diagnosis and to the understanding of the mechanisms responsible for joint damage, functional impairment, and deformity has not been sufficiently appreciated.

This volume covers two broad fields. Firstly, the radiologic appearances of various disorders other than rheumatoid arthritis that serve to illustrate the basic changes which may involve the soft tissues are described. This aspect of the work is not intended to be a complete survey, and some lesions which have been of particular interest to the authors receive more detailed attention than do others. The soft tissues may be displaced by a dislocation or subluxation, the soft tissue planes may be obscured by interstitial edema and hemorrhage, and occasionally abnormal soft tissue shadows are due to fibrous, fatty, or vascular proliferation. The radiologic appearances of such common lesions as ruptured muscles and distended joints, tendon sheaths and bursae, are characteristic.

However, the soft tissue changes associated with rheumatoid arthritis are the principal concern of the authors. This disease is quite common and, apart from trauma, is the most likely disorder to affect those structures which are lined by synovium, ie, the joints, tendon sheaths, and bursae. The radiologic changes in the soft tissue produced by involvement of the more important of these structures are illustrated. Added emphasis is given by the inclusion of contrast studies, which often show both the unexpected extent of some of these lesions and the bizarre forms they may take.

The authors feel that a record of their experience in the interpretation of soft tissue lesions could lead to a wider appreciation of the scope of radiologic interpretation. The standard of rheumatologic practice is raised by challenging and detailed radiologic reports. Thus, this monograph has been written to further the appreciation of soft tissue involvement in the rheumatic diseases.

Acknowledgments

This volume represents the combined efforts of a rheumatologist and a radiologist working toward the common goal of improving the radiologic recognition of arthritic disease. We are most grateful for the help we have received from many sources. Associate Professor Charles Begg and his staff of the Radiology Department, Dunedin Public Hospital and radiographers of the Hutt area (Mr. C. K. Kelsey, Miss M. Jennings, Mrs. M. Gordon, Miss H. Kraus, Miss M. Desborough, Mrs. C. Sache, and Miss Janet M. Robertson) have all helped and contributed to this work. Mr. Kelsey established the soft tissue techniques which have been used in this study.

Dr. Patricia Cairney (Hutt Hospital) and Professor J. B. Blennerhassett (University of Otago Medical School) have made their departments available for the postmortem studies. The reproduction of radiographs and other illustrations is due to the expertise of Mr. Rees B. Sparke at Wellington Hospital and to Mr. B. P. Connor and Mr. D. V. Weston at Dunedin. At the Hutt Hospital Mr. G. R. Laurenson and Mr. C. J. Bossley (orthopedic surgeons) and Dr. J. Moore Tweed and Dr. B. L. J. Treadwell (rheumatologists) are thanked for their interest and support.

Miss Pamela Tunnage, Dunedin, has patiently carried out the typing of the manuscript.

Financial support from the Medical Research Council of New Zealand is gratefully acknowledged.

W. J. W. is particularly grateful to his mentor, Dr. O. C.

Moller, who first introduced him to the radiology of the soft tissues and to the work of Albert Ferguson. This set the stage for the whole study. He also wishes to record his gratitude to his present partner, Dr. John Roberts, who made this work possible by allowing him the opportunity to pursue and develop this study which became a lifelong interest.

Professor W. P. Gowland and Professor W. E. Adams were our teachers in the Anatomy Department of the University of Otago and we are grateful for their superb training and guidance.

Finally, we should like to thank the Editors of the following journals for their permission to reproduce material: Journal of Bone and Joint Surgery, Arthritis and Rheumatism, Annals of the Rheumatic Diseases, British Journal of Radiology, Journal of the Canadian Association of Radiologists, Australian Radiology, Annals of Internal Medicine, and the New Zealand Medical Journal.

Acknowledgments

Contents

Contents

CHAPTER 1

Introduction

RADIOGRAPHIC SOFT TISSUE TECHNIQUES

Soft tissue structures can best be demonstrated by specialized techniques; however, in most cases the soft tissues and bone details are required at the same time.

Mention must be made of mammography, as the present techniques developed from this method. Egan's work was followed here (6). A Conrad 300 mA unit was used, and was modified by a special switch to reduce the kV by 20 kV on the 300 mA setting only. This gave a kV range from 20 to 100 kV in steps of 2 kV. Filters were removed from the tube and a long extension cylinder of 3-inch diameter was used. A craniocaudal and mediolateral view of each breast was taken.

However, unlike Egan's description, we used a double-film technique. An Agfa Mammography T3 film is placed over an Agfa Industrial D7 film. The latter film is the faster one and shows the denser structures and the retromammary fat. Average exposure factors for this examination are 300 mA, 96.5 cm, 6 seconds. Craniocaudal view 30 kV, mediolateral 32 kV.

It seemed a pity that other uses could not be made of this low kV and fine grain film technique. Using the mammography technique with distance and time reduced, glass fragments can be demonstrated in areas such as the lips, nose, and eyelids. A further use is in de Quervain's disease. The space-taking tendon sheath mass is easily demonstrated deforming the cutis line. The posteroanterior views of both wrists must be taken, as a control in some cases and for demonstration of bilateral cases in others (44).

Would it be possible to produce comparable results using industrial film and factors available to most radiographers? Using industrial film, normal kV and mA, and times suitable to the film, it was possible to produce good bone as well as soft tissue detail. It was found that Agfa Industrial D7 film had similar characteristics to Kodak type M, but required half the exposure time. Using industrial film and factors in the region of 100 mA, 1.5 seconds, and 76 cm distance, good quality radiographs of the extremities could be obtained.

Standard nonscreen film still has an important part to play in general radiography. The time factor for this film is 0.75 seconds. Standard nonscreen film has been used for lateral views of the knees with an 8:1 moving grid. Time here is 3 seconds with Agfa-Osray M3 nonscreen film.

This section has not covered all types of soft tissue examinations, nor does it imply that the foregoing are the only or best methods of demonstrating soft tissue. The mammography technique gives the best result where the best possible soft tissue definition is required. There are many instances where such fine differentiation is not required, and then industrial film and normal mA and kV give adequate results.

In all cases in which industrial film is used, it is necessary to give twice the normal standard development time. Where standard nonscreen film is used, the normal development time is satisfactory.

Summary of Film and Factors [Kelsey C. K.]

Agfa Industrial D7 film:
  76 cm distance, 100 mA, 1-second exposure, 40 to 56 kV
  Manual development: 70 F, 5.5 minutes
Agfa-Osray M3 Nonscreen:
  76 cm distance, 50 mA, 0.5-second exposure, 40 to 56 kV
  Automatic processor (3.5-minute cycle)
Agfa-Osray M3 Nonscreen:
  For shoulders and knees with 8:1 moving grid.
  76 cm distance, 100 mA, 3-seconds exposure, 54 to 64 kV
  Automatic processor (3.5-minute cycle)

It is important to remember that the best results are obtained when the film is processed by hand. Some departments have given up hand processing and thus will have to modify their techniques and film used. Some mammography-type film is now made to pass through the automatic processer, but this is only second best.

Lastly, but most important of all, a radiographer is required who is both interested and artistic. The results should please and delight all those introduced to this method.

XERORADIOGRAPHY

Xeroradiography is the science of recording radiographic images electronically on a charged selenium plate. Negatively charged powder (toner) is dusted over the plate and it adheres to the positively charged image. A sheet of paper is then placed over the plate and receives a positive charge. This positively charged paper attracts powder from the plate, forming a direct positive image. The print is then fixed by heat for a few seconds to form the permanent image.

Xeroradiograms have an excellent resolving power at all levels of contrast. A unique feature of the system is the "edge effect." Where there is discontinuity in density, the margins become exaggerated, i.e., there is edge enhancement. This is due to the heaping up of the powder at the boundary. This edge contrast increases the visibility of any vascular or fibrous structure lying in the soft tissues (46).

Now where there is a very marked difference in contrast, as in an area immediately surrounding a heavily calcified area, there will be a white area where the detail is lost. This is the so-called halo effect, or, as one author calls it, the tono steel (22).

Xeroradiography can be used for the study of bones and joints. The technique suggested incorporates the use of a high kV [120 kVP (kilovoltage peak)] and low mA. The soft tissues are said to be better shown in xeroradiography than in conventional radiography, but the lack of fine resolution may reduce this advantage. The authors themselves have had no experience with this method.

The Fascial Planes

In the normal extremity the junction between the fat and the deep fascia is seen as a clearly defined interface in the soft tissue radiograph. This has been called the fat–fascia interface. Fatty planes are also present between the muscles in the limbs. These represent the perimuscular fat that surrounds each muscle and which allow the muscles to move one upon the other. Fatty planes are especially prominent in the thigh but are present in all areas of the body.

On occasion, particularly in obese patients, one can define fine fibrous connective tissue strands running from the deep fascia out to the cutis line. These may be interconnected by further strands that run in the long axis of the limb. These fine strands contain the neurovascular bundles to the skin. They are best seen in the soft tissues under the heel.

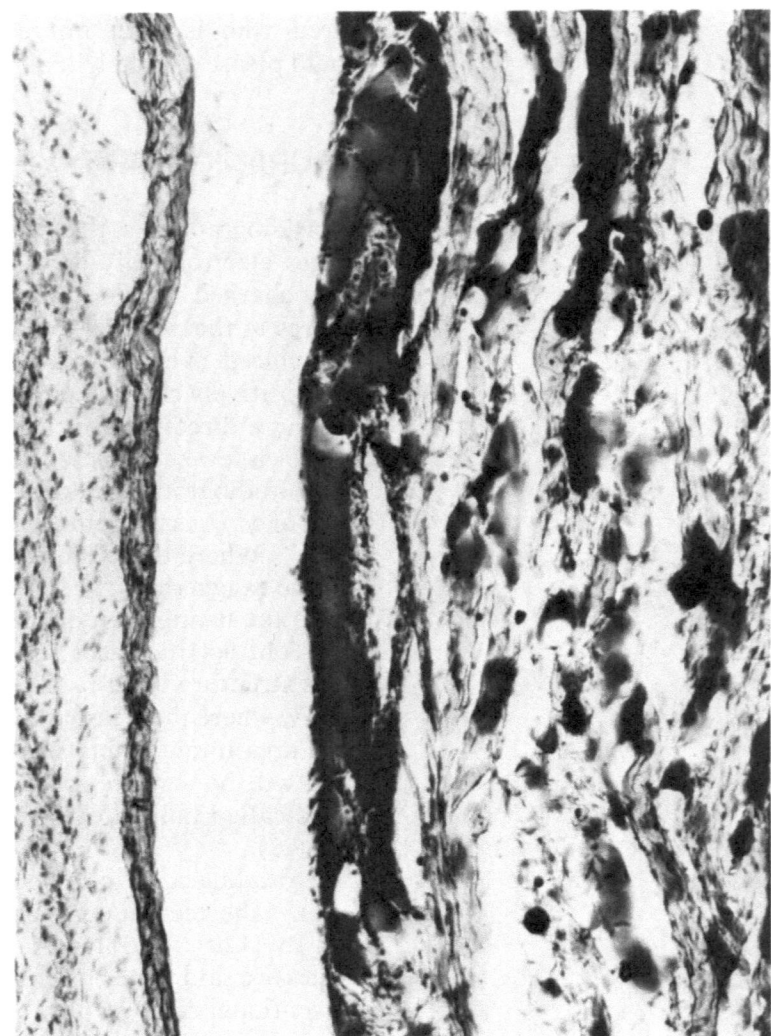

Fig. 1-1. A longitudinal section through the subdeltoid extension of the subacromial bursa to illustrate the extrasynovial fat clothing the superficial surface. H & E, ×135.

The presence of extrasynovial fat about bursae and joint capsules produces lines of demarcation in the soft tissue radiograph (Fig. 1-1). Alteration in the normal contours of these translucent envelopes is often the earliest evidence of distension by an effusion.

Edema

Edema in the limbs causes thickening of the fine connective tissue strands that run from the deep fascia to the skin. Radiologically this is seen as a coarse network in the subcutaneous fat (Fig. 1-2). Edema produces this pattern whatever the underlying cause. The radiologic changes associated with edema can thus be reproduced by injecting normal sa-

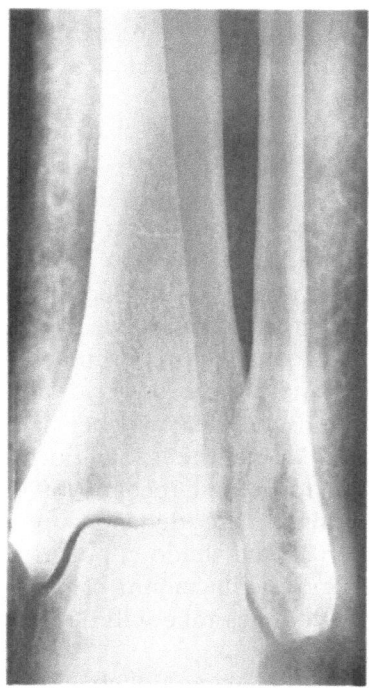

Fig. 1-2. Edema causes thickening of the fine connective tissue strands that run from the deep fascia to the skin. Other strands run in the long axis of the limb and are thickened also.

line into the subcutaneous tissues. A similar pattern can be seen when one of the soluble iodine-containing contrast media is used in combination with hyaluronidase (Fig. 1-3) (9). Edema in the intermuscular fat produces disruption and then loss of the fatty planes. There is an associated increase in the diameter of the limb, which is best appreciated by comparison with views of the other limb.

One of the commonest causes of edema is venous stasis resulting from a thrombophlebitis or phlebothrombosis. A more localized form can be seen involving the soft tissues overlying an osteomyelitis.

Lymphatic stasis can also produce edema, with thickening of the cutis line. Other conditions such as cellulitis, erysipelas, erythema nodosum, and erythema induratum all produce edema in the subcutaneous tissues and cutis line. These lesions may be differentiated by considering the total clinical picture. Erythema nodosum and induratum, for example, produce a localized soft tissue change, in contrast to the more widespread changes of venous and lymphatic stasis. In contrast, the edema seen with deep vein thrombosis and in the early stages of an acute osteomyelitis involves both muscle and subcutaneous tissues. According to Frantzell (9), similar widening of the muscle mass rarely occurs in uncomplicated lymphatic stasis.

Hemorrhage

With trauma, hematoma formation is quite a common finding in the limb. Hematoma produces a dense homogeneous mass in the subcutaneous tissues that becomes continuous with both the cutis line and the deep fascia. It is a mass lesion and thus produces an increase in the diameter of the limb.

When the hematoma is in the muscle layers, the fatty intermuscular layers are disrupted or lost. There is an increase in the volume of the muscle. This is the soft tissue finding prior to the development of myositis ossificans.

Tendinitis Calcarea

Tendinitis calcarea is commonly seen about the shoulder joint, but may be seen about any joint of the appendicular skeleton. In the acute form the calcification may appear as cloudy, ill-defined areas or as cloudy areas between denser and better-defined deposits (Fig. 1-4). In the chronic form the area of calcification is usually homogeneous, dense, and well defined. In the acute cases there is edema about the area of calcification and this can act as a space-taking lesion. When the supraspinatus tendon is involved the swelling can displace the humeral head in a caudal direction. On occasions a

Introduction

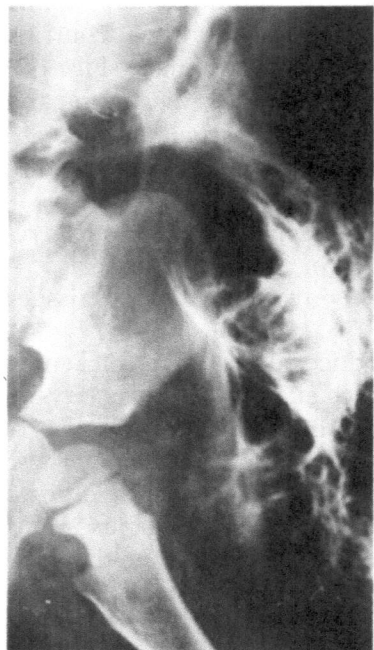

Fig. 1-3. A similar pattern to that of edema is seen when hypaque is used in combination with hyaluronidase in subcutaneous injections.

sympathetic effusion in the related joint may be recognized. This may present an acute arthritis. As the lesion settles down the effusion is absorbed (40).

The Synovial Mass

Since the synovial membrane, synovial fluid, edema fluid, and melon-seed bodies all have the same density they cannot be differentiated in the plain film and are best considered as a single synovial complex. Only an arthrogram allows one to determine whether a synovial mass consists predominantly of synovial fluid, thickened synovial membrane, or of rice and melon-seed bodies. Such a synovial complex will act as a mass lesion. It will displace the cutis line, the fascia–fat interface, and the muscle layers. The radiologic recognition of tissue changes in rheumatoid arthritis thus depends upon two simple signs: an abnormal soft tissue shadow, outlined by translucent extrasynovial fat, and displacement of other tissues. The particular form these changes take will depend upon the anatomic structures affected.

The ulnar bursa proved to be a suitable synovial structure for the experimental correlation of soft tissue swelling and radiologic change. Water was injected through a 21-gauge needle introduced percutaneously about 3 cm above the lower

Fig. 1-4. Calcification in the supraspinatus tendon. In this section of a surgical specimen the irregular deposition of calcium is apparent. von Kossa, × 30.

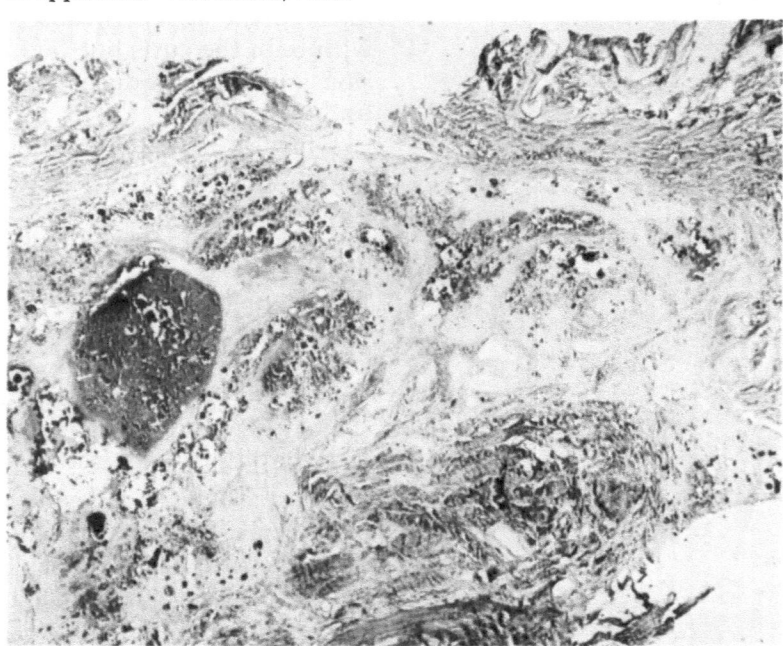

wrist crease into the ulnar bursa at postmortem. A point medial to the tendon of palmaris longus was used, as this was an easy surface marking to identify. The ideal volume of water for distending this structure was found to be 3 ml followed by 3 ml of hypaque 50 percent. Five ml of each fluid was found to rupture the bursa. Plain films were taken prior to the introduction of the needle and the water (Fig. 1-5A). The hypaque injection was a check that the ulnar bursa was injected and filled (Fig. 1-5B and C) (45).

The following soft tissue signs were subsequently noted in the radiographs.

1. A measurable increase in the thickness of the soft tissues ventral to the lower end of the radius.
2. A reduction in the thickness of the layer of extrasynovial fat over pronator quadratus. The length of this visible fatty layer was also reduced.
3. The fat plane between the tendons of flexor profundus digitorum and flexor sublimus digitorum was obliterated.
4. The extrasynovial fat about the ulnar bursa could be seen when the bursa was outlined by contrast. It formed a thin crescent about the proximal pole of the distended bursa, and intersected at right angles the intermuscular fatty plane over pronator quadratus.

In order to test the hypothesis that part of the fat seen on the ventral aspect of pronator quadratus was in continuity with that surrounding the bursa, views of the wrist were taken in full extension, full flexion, and in the semiflexed and semiextended positions. In extreme extension of the wrist, the bellies of flexor sublimus digitorum and flexor profundus digitorum moved peripherally, and the fat about the ulnar bursa was also seen to shift to the lower margin of pronator quadratus in the form of a flat, truncated cone (Fig. 1-5D). At postmortem the free mobility of this fat pad, which allows movement between the pronator quadratus and the flexor tendons, can be easily demonstrated.

Intrasynovial fat deposits may be visible in the soft tissue radiograph. Berens and Lin (3) noted soft tissue masses that contained areas of translucency and which were, in all probability, fatty deposits. Such deposits may be very conspicuous in the synovium in the condition of lipoma arborescens (10), and can be responsible for the translucent areas which may be seen within the synovial mass in patients with rheumatoid arthritis.

The lipid content of synovial fluid itself may be of radiologic significance and may produce a water–fat interface. Kim and Cohen (17) have discussed the synovial fluid fatty acid composition in patients with rheumatoid arthritis.

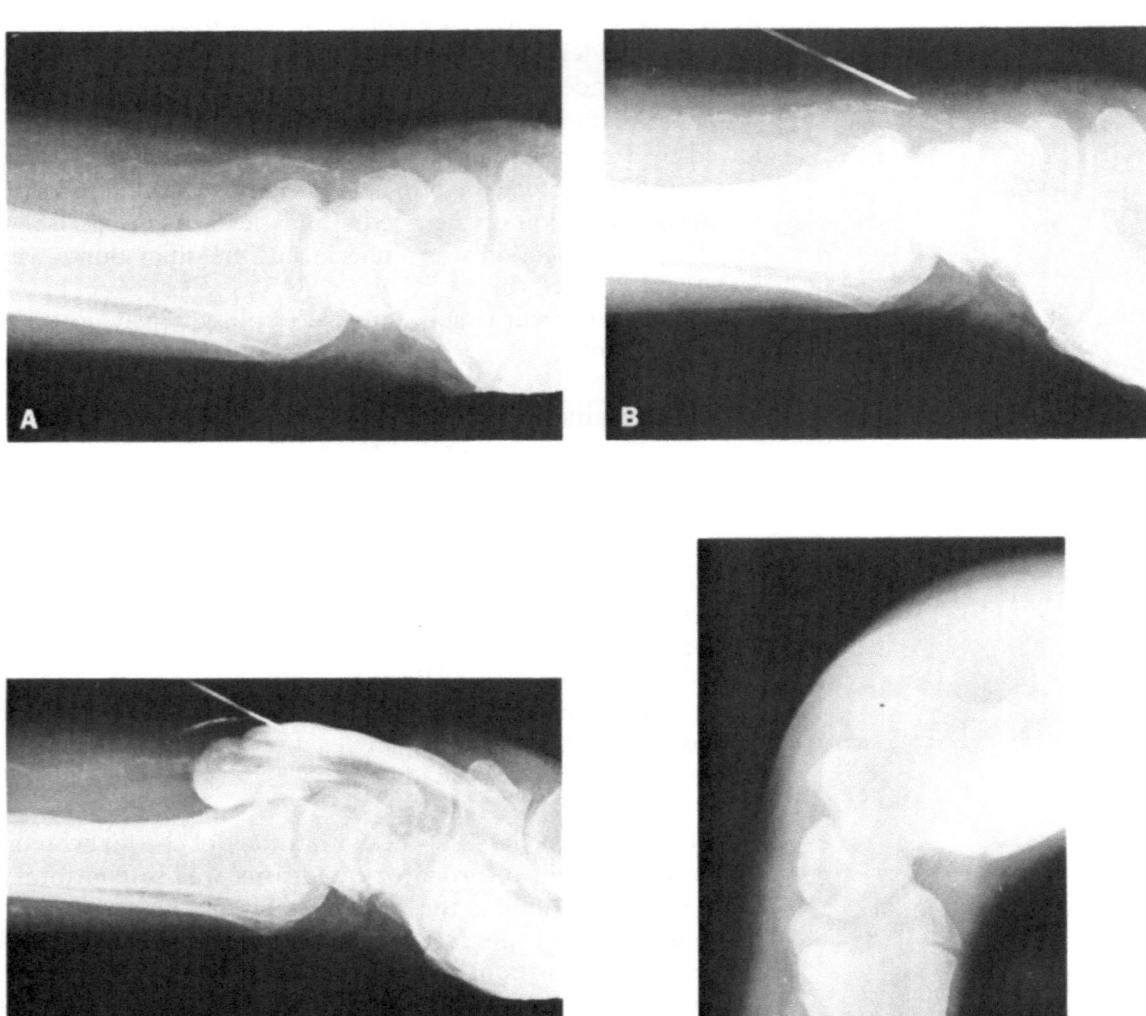

Fig. 1-5. A. Lateral soft tissue view of wrist prior to insertion of butterfly needle at postmortem examination. **B.** Lateral view of wrist following injection of 5 ml of water into the ulnar bursa. The change in size and shape of the extrasynovial fat on the pronator quadratus is well shown. The loss of fat between the tendons of flexor profundus digitorum and the muscle and tendons of flexor sublimus digitorum may also be noted. The soft tissues are increased in thickness on the ventral aspect of the radius. **C.** A further lateral view of the wrist after additional injection of 3 ml of hypaque into the ulnar bursa. This acts as a check on the position of the butterfly needle. The extrasynovial fat about the proximal pole of the ulnar bursa can be seen. **D.** Lateral view of wrist in hyperextension. The fat about the ulnar bursa lies at the lower margin of pronator quadratus muscle in the form of a truncated cone. (*From Weston: J Can Assoc Radiol 24:282, 1973.*)

Bone Erosions

Erosions in bone represent the aggressive margin of the synovial mass. Thus, these erosions outline the advancement of the soft tissue changes. In the active phase erosions may be poorly demarcated. As the acute phase settles the erosions tend to heal and become marginated. Rarely, complete filling of the erosions can take place.

Enlarged Lymph Glands

Ragan (30) noted that in about 50 percent of cases of rheumatoid arthritis there is a generalized lymphadenopathy. It is possible to show these enlarged glands quite clearly when industrial film is used. Enlarged supratrochlear glands and axillary glands in particular have been reported (42, 43).

Soft Tissue Changes in Rheumatoid Arthritis

Ferguson (7) stated: "Roentgenograms for the detection of rheumatoid arthritis should depict the soft tissue shadows as clearly as the bone shadows. In rheumatoid arthritis, particularly in the early stages, there are changes in the soft tissues at the joint; and changes in the relative density of bone and soft tissues which are important and which can be detected only if the soft tissues are clearly pictured."

Various factors contribute to the final radiologic picture. The synovial tissues are affected by a number of pathologic changes that contribute to the soft tissue appearances visible on radiologic examination. To a greater or lesser degree, cellular proliferation and infiltration, increased vascularity, interstitial edema, fibrinoid deposition, and, particularly, exudation of synovial fluid contribute to the increased bulk of the affected tissues. In addition, rice and melon-seed bodies and intrasynovial fatty masses may contribute to the increased bulk of the synovium.

The proliferation of the synovium may be exuberant. The synovial villus is normally an inconspicuous structure of variable form (Fig. 1-6A–C). When involved by the rheumatoid process, however, the villi become enlarged and swollen (Fig. 1-6D) and groups of villi may form large, complex, pedunculated structures which, when floated out in saline after synovectomy, resemble masses of seaweed (27). The synoviocytes lining involved joints, bursae, or tendon sheaths enlarge and proliferate. Fibrinoid material commonly is deposited both on the surface and within the deeper tissues of the synovial membrane. An infiltrate of chronic inflammatory cells is always present and is sometimes sufficient to give the impression that the interstitial tissues are choked with cells. The increased blood flow to the involved joint is reflected in the in-

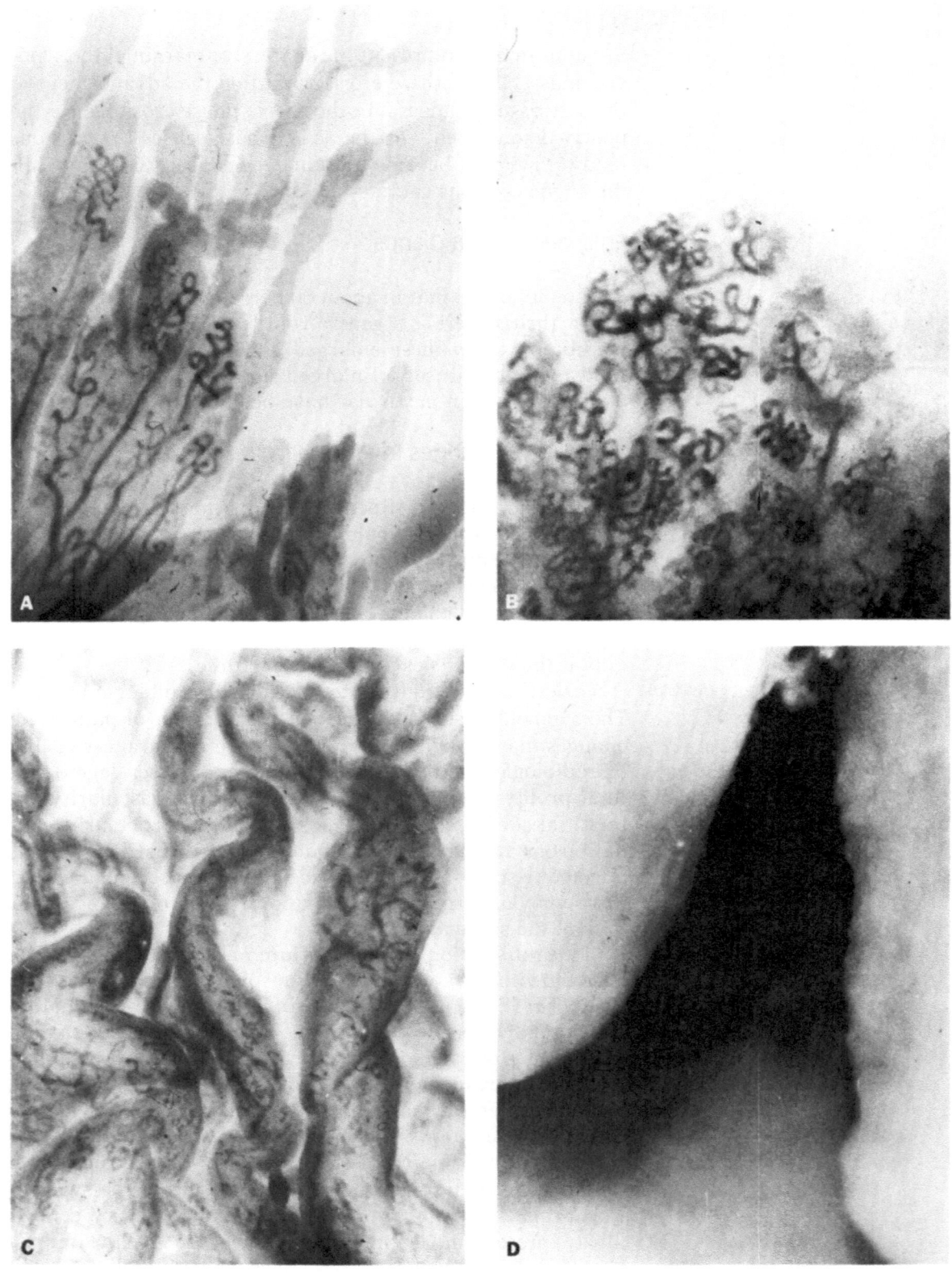

Fig. 1-6.

creased numbers of synovial blood vessels seen histologically, in the increased clearance rates of substances such as phenolsulphonphthalein (25), and in the results of actual blood flow measurements (26).

This exuberant proliferating mass of synovial tissue does not remain confined to the synovial space. Destruction of cartilage and adjacent bone is followed by the invasion and replacement of these structures by granulation tissue. Disruption of the soft tissue integument may lead to sacculation of the synovial lining.

Radiologically, the bone erosions form one apparently definite peripheral boundary to the soft tissue mass. Histologically, however, the proliferating granulation tissue extends beyond this radiologic boundary and into the exposed trabecular system of the underlying bone. Joint damage found at surgery is always in excess of the radiologic changes and, even in the absence of radiologic change, the articular cartilage may be quite extensively damaged.

Within the tendon sheaths rheumatoid granulation tissue may mechanically interfere with tendon action, and may extend along the vincular vessels to invade the tendons and cause damage which may lead to tendon rupture (38). The pathologic changes within the walls of involved bursae are similar. Granulation tissue may extend from involved bursae and from subcutaneous rheumatoid nodules into the underlying bone producing erosion (Fig. 1-7).

The main factor, however, resulting in swollen joints, tendon sheaths, and bursae, is usually fluid accumulation. The exact nature of the disturbance of fluid exchange across the synoviocapillary barrier has been only partly defined (29). Some factors, however, have been well established. Capillary permeability is increased and this is reflected in increased concentration of the protein constituents of the synovial fluid (32) and in altered permeability to isotopically labelled proteins (39). Although the colloidal osmotic pressure of a pathologic synovial effusion is increased, the osmotic gradient does not favor fluid passage into the joint (20). In contrast, the passage of crystalloids through the inflamed synovial membrane may actually be depressed (33, 35). Of practical importance is the level to which the hydrostatic pressure

---

Fig. 1-6. A. Vascular leaf-shaped villi. The avascular elongated processes arising from these villi are secondary villi. Evans blue, oblique light, × 80. **B.** A vascular fan-shaped villus. One of a series arising from the circumpatellar pad and directed toward the patella. Oblique light, × 80. **C.** Villous folds from the lower posterior surface of the suprapatellar bursa. Oblique light, × 80. **D.** The villi become enlarged and swollen when involved by the rheumatoid process. No vascular network is visible beneath the granular opaque surface. Oblique light, × 80. (*From Palmer: Arthritis Rheum 10:451, 1967.*)

Introduction

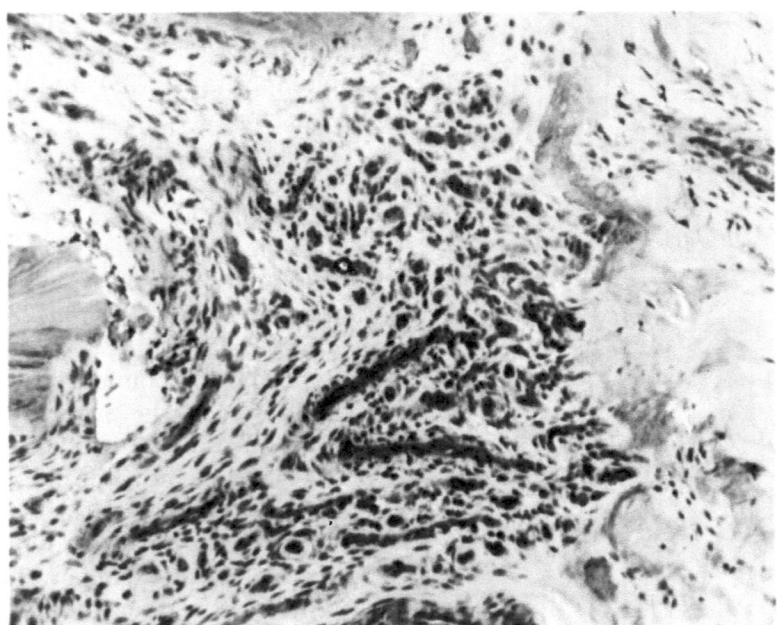

Fig. 1-7. Rheumatoid inflammatory tissue invading the trabecular system of the os calcis from the retrocalcareal bursa.

Fig. 1-8. Pressure-volume relationships in rheumatoid knees containing effusions. The hydrostatic pressure may be quite high. Graphs constructed from measurements of hydrostatic pressure undertaken during step-wise aspiration from knee joints. *(From Palmer and Myers: Arthritis Rheum 11:745, 1968.)*

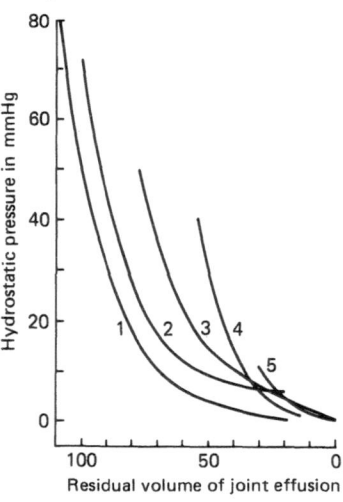

of an effusion may rise (Fig. 1-8). Measurement of this parameter has been largely restricted to the knee joint. Such studies have shown that even at rest the intraarticular hydrostatic pressure of an involved knee joint may be unexpectedly high—certainly as high as 80 mm Hg (29)—and that physical maneuvers designed to place the joint under load, such as knee bending, may increase the pressure to levels which may actually produce capsular rupture (6). Such increases in hydrostatic pressure are no doubt related to complications which may involve the rheumatoid joint such as synovial sacculation, capsular rupture, and deformity (28).

A further factor of importance in determining the actual configuration of a joint, tendon sheath, or bursa that contains an effusion is related to the possibility that some alteration in the compliance of the capsule and surrounding tissues has occurred. It has been shown that capsular compliance is reduced in older patients with rheumatoid arthritis. Furthermore, some temporary alteration in compliance can be induced in a normal knee joint simply by distending it with saline beyond its elastic limit (24). Localized areas of the joint integument doubtless may be more affected than others, and this may contribute to unexpected radiologic configurations. Compliance may be defined as the change in intraarticular volume per unit change in intraarticular pressure (dV/dP). This concept is possibly more readily grasped conceptually than that introduced by Jayson and Dixon (13, 14). These authors used the term elastance to document changes in cap-

Soft Tissues of the Extremities

sular elasticity, and defined this in reciprocal terms as a change in pressure per unit change in volume (dP/dV). Defined in this way, these authors have shown elastance to be increased in rheumatoid joints.

Rheumatoid Subcutaneous Nodules

Rheumatoid nodules characterize the more severe cases of the disease and are associated with circulating IgM rheumatoid factors. Recognition is thus of some prognostic importance. Although usually found over the dorsal surface of the ulna below the olecranon, these lesions may occur in other rather odd locations including the occipital region, the subcutaneous tissues of the fingers, the heels, and superficially to the Achilles tendon. In size and number they vary from an inconspicuous seedlike structure within the subcutaneous tissues to large multicentered lesions. Histologically the earliest lesions are thought to be based on a vasculitis (37). The fully developed nodule has a characteristic histologic appearance comprised of a central necrotic zone, an intermediate cellular zone of histiocytes arranged en palisade, and a peripheral zone composed of chronic inflammatory cells and fibroblasts. Erosive changes occasionally involve the underlying bone.

Lymphatic Involvement in Rheumatoid Arthritis

Reticuloendothelial involvement is now considered to be present to some extent in the majority of cases of rheumatoid arthritis, although the reported incidence has varied widely, reflecting the difficulty in deciding what constituted a "significant lymphadenopathy" (36). Pathologic studies have demonstrated structural changes in the lymphatic system in rheumatoid arthritis (23). The histologic changes are nonspecific and consist of follicular hyperplasia, reticuloendothelial activity, and some connective tissue proliferation.

Radiologically this "rheumatoid lymphadenopathy" has been demonstrated by lymphangiography (31), but soft tissue radiography may demonstrate lymph node enlargement quite adequately, especially if the radiographs are taken on industrial film using the mammography technique. The demonstration of lymph node enlargement (Fig. 1-9) is useful additional evidence of an inflammatory arthritis involving the adjacent joints (2). Sometimes, however, the lymphadenopathy may be of sinister significance, and the radiologist should be aware of the association between rheumatoid arthritis and various reticuloses (11).

Any functional disturbance of the lymphatic channels would be of significance. The rate at which contrast material leaves a joint has been used as a measure of absorptive capac-

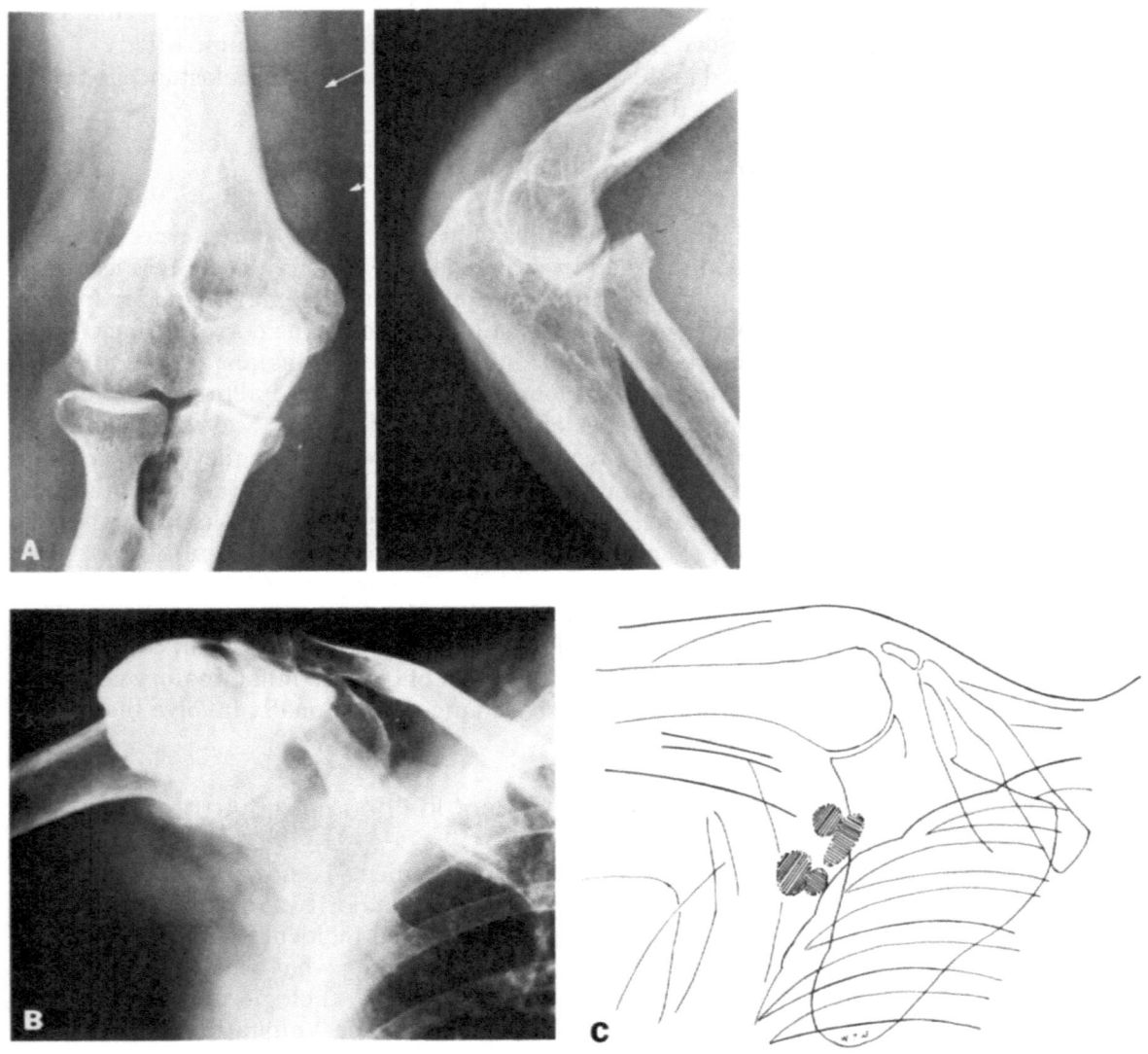

Fig. 1-9. A. Anterior and lateral projections of the right elbow. Rheumatoid arthritis is present with a well-marked synovial change. Two enlarged supratrochlear lymph glands are noted (arrows). **B.** Arthrogram of shoulder with contrast in subdeltoid bursa due to a defect in the rotator cuff. The enlarged glands are visible in the axilla. **C.** Line diagram of plain film. Hatched areas represent enlarged lymphatic glands. (*Fig. 1-9A: From Weston: Australas Radiol 12:260, 1968. Fig. 1-9B, C: From Weston: Australas Radiol 15:55, 1971.*)

ity of the synovial membrane (34). Adkins and Davies (1) showed that lymphatic drainage played little part in the absorption of a contrast agent, uroselectan B, from normal rabbit joints, and lymphatic filling has never been observed in any of the many hundreds of postmortem arthrograms which have been carried out in the course of this study.

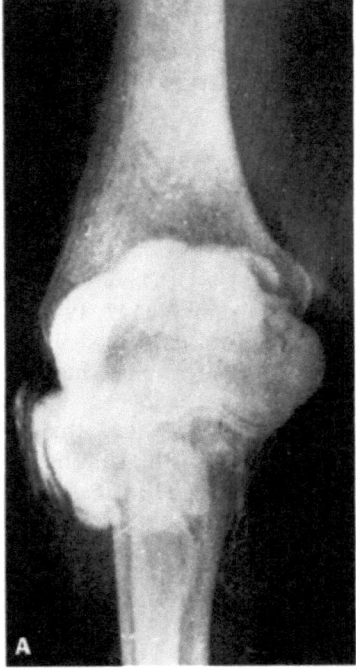
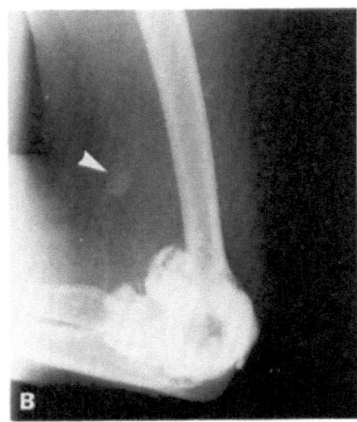

Fig. 1-10: **A.** Anteroposterior projection of the elbow joint. The enlarged synovial cavity is well shown. A small amount of opaque medium was extravasated into the soft tissues on the lateral aspect of the joint at the injection site. Numerous filling defects are noted in the joint cavity. The filled lymphatic vessels are seen on the medial aspect of the joint. **B.** The lymphatic vessels are well demonstrated arising from the ventral aspect of the joint. The supratrochlear lymph nodes have also been outlined (arrow). (*From Weston: Australas Radiol 13:368, 1968.*)

During positive contrast arthrography of joints involved by rheumatoid arthritis, however, lymphatic filling has been observed in about 20 percent of cases (Fig. 1-10), but has not been observed in conjunction with arthrograms undertaken for internal derangement of knee joints, nor with other joints investigated for complaints other than rheumatoid arthritis (41).

Lewin and Mulhern (19) reviewed the literature on lymphatic visualization during arthrography. Their experience and that of other observers was that lymphatic visualization during contrast arthrography was a reliable indication of the presence of rheumatoid disease of the joint.

The principal lymphatic channels draining the limbs have been reported as appearing normal (31), but occasionally, when diffuse edema involves an extremity affected by rheumatoid disease, lymphatic drainage may be obstructed (15). Haage (12), however, has reported lymphatic filling during arthrography in cases of trauma to a joint. It would seem that the lymphatic system plays an extended role in the drainage of joints involved by rheumatoid disease; but it should be noted that Kuhns (18) found obliterations of synovial lymphatics in "atrophic" arthritis.

References

1. Adkins EWO, Davies DV: Absorption from the joint cavity. QJ Exp Physiol 30:147, 1940
2. Baggenstoss AH, Rosenberg EF: Visceral lesions associated with chronic infections (rheumatoid) arthritis. Arch Pathol 35:503, 1943
3. Berens DL, Lin R-K: Roentgen Diagnosis of Rheumatoid Arthritis. Springfield, Ill, Thomas, 1969, p 180
4. Bywaters EGL: Heel lesions of rheumatoid arthritis. Ann Rheum Dis 13:42, 1954
5. Bywaters EGL: In Carter M (ed): Radiological Aspects of Rheumatoid Arthritis. Amsterdam, Excerpta Medica, 1963, pp 3–259
6. Egan RL: Mammography. Springfield, Ill, Thomas, 1964, pp 3–70
7. Ferguson AB: Roentgenographic features of rheumatoid arthritis. Bone Joint Surg, 18:297, 1936 (Old Series)
8. Forrester DM, Nesson JW: The Radiology of Joint Disease. Philadelphia, Saunders, 1973, pp 3–463
9. Frantzell A: Radiology of Muscles, Skin, and Subcutaneous Tissues. Modern Trends in Diagnostic Radiology. Second series. London, Butterworth, 1953, pp 239–250
10. Gardner DL: Pathology of the Connective Tissue Diseases. London, Arnold, 1965, pp 403–405
11. Goldenberg GJ, Paraskevas F, Israels LG: The association of rheumatoid arthritis with plasma cell and lymphocytic neoplasms. Arthritis Rheum 12:569, 1969
12. Haage H: Die Arthrographie des Sprunggelenkes. Radiologe 5:137, 1967
13. Jayson MIV, Dixon AStJ: Intra-articular pressure in rheumatoid arthritis of the knee. I. Pressure changes during passive joint distension. Ann Rheum Dis 29:261, 1970
14. Jayson MIV, Dixon AStJ: Intra-articular pressure in rheumatoid arthritis of the knee. III. Pressure change during joint use. Ann Rheum Dis 29:401, 1970
15. Kalliomaki JL, Vastamaki M: Chronic diffuse edema of the rheumatoid hand. A sign of local lymphatic involvement. Ann Rheum Dis 27:167, 1968
16. Kelsey CK: Personal communication page 2b
17. Kim IC, Cohen AS: Synovial fluid fatty acid composition in patients with rheumatoid arthritis, gout, and degenerative joint disease. Proc Soc Exp Biol Med 123:77, 1966
18. Kuhns JG: Lymphatic drainage of joints. Arch Surg 27:345, 1933
19. Lewin JR, Mulhern LM: Lymphatic visualisation during contrast arthrography of the knee. Radiology 103:577, 1972

20. Lipson RL, Baldes EJ, Anderson JA, et al: Osmotic pressure gradients and joint effusions. Arthritis Rheum 8:29, 1965

21. Martel W, Hayes JT, Duff IF: The pattern of bone erosion in the hand and wrist in rheumatoid arthritis. Radiology 84:204, 1965

22. Morrison AM: Xeroradiography. Shadows 17:19, 1974

23. Motulsky AG, Weinberg S, Saphir O, et al: Lymph nodes in rheumatoid arthritis. Arch Intern Med 90:660, 1952

24. Myers DB, Palmer DG: Capsular compliance and pressure volume relationships in normal and arthritic knees. J Bone Joint Surg [Br] 54:710, 1972

25. Nakamura R, Asai H, Sonozaki H, et al: Phenolsulphonphthalein clearance from the knee joint in normal and pathological states. Ann Rheum Dis 26:246, 1967

26. Onge RA, St, Dick WC: Some applications of gamma-emitting radioisotopes in rheumatology. In Hill AGS (ed): Modern Trends in Rheumatology, Volume 2. Glasgow, Bell and Bain, 1971

27. Palmer DG: Synovial villi. An examination of these structures within the anterior compartment of the knee and metacarpophalangeal joints. Arthritis Rheum 10:451, 1967

28. Palmer DG: Dynamics of joint disruption. NZ Med J 78:166, 1973

29. Palmer DG, Myers DB: Some observations of joint effusions. Arthritis Rheum 11:745, 1968

30. Ragan C: (1966). Clinical picture of rheumatoid arthritis. In Hollander JL (ed): Arthritis and Allied Conditions, 7th ed. Philadelphia, Lea & Febiger, 1966, pp 215–216

31. Robertson MDJ, Hart FD, White WF, et al: Rheumatoid lymphadenopathy. Ann Rheum Dis 27:253, 1968

32. Ropes MW, Bauer W: Synovial Fluid Changes in Joint Disease. Cambridge, Mass, Harvard Univ Press, 1953, p 39

33. Ropes MW, Muller AF, Bauer W: The entrance of glucose and other sugars into joints. Arthritis Rheum 3:496, 1960

34. Sallis JG, Perry BJ: Absorption from the synovial cavity in rabbits and cats. The influence of different environments and drugs. S Afr J Med Sci 32:83, 1967

35. Scholer JF, Lee PR, Polley HF: The absorption of heavy water and radioactive sodium from the knee joint of normal persons and patients with rheumatoid arthritis. Arthritis Rheum 2:426, 1959

36. Short CL, Bauer W, Reynolds WE: Rheumatoid Arthritis. Cambridge, Mass, Harvard Univ Press, 1957, p 311

37. Sokoloff L, McCluskey RT, Bunim JJ: Vascularity of the early subcutaneous nodule of rheumatoid arthritis. Arch Pathol 55:475, 1953

38. Tarr KH: Spontaneous rupture of tendons in rheumatoid arthritis. NZ Med J 79:651, 1974

39. Weiss TE, Maxfield WS, Murison PJ, et al: Iodinated human serum albumin (I[131]) localization studies of rheumatoid arthritis joints by scintillation scanning. Arthritis Rheum 8:976, 1965

40. Weston WJ: Tendinitis calcarea of the extensor origin of the elbow with effusion of the joint. Acta Radiol (Stockh) 54:120, 1960

Introduction

41. Weston WJ: Lymphatic filling during positive contrast arthography in rheumatoid arthritis. Australas Radiol 13:368, 1969
42. Weston WJ: Enlarged supratrochlear lymphatic glands in rheumatoid arthritis. Australas Radiol 12:260, 1968
43. Weston WJ: Enlarged axillary glands in rheumatoid arthritis. Australas Radiol 15:55, 1971
44. Weston WJ: De Quervain's disease. Stenosing fibrous tendovaginitis at the radial styloid process. Br J Radiol 40:446, 1967
45. Weston WJ: The soft tissue signs of the enlarged ulnar bursa in rheumatoid arthritis. J Can Assoc Radiol 24:282, 1973
46. Wolf JN: Xeroradiography of the Breast. Presented at the 7th National Cancer Conference, Los Angeles, September 27–29, 1972

CHAPTER 2

The Shoulder Region

In 1934 Codman (3) described rupture of the supraspinatus tendon and other lesions in and about the subacromial bursa. The most recent publication of his work is still the best reference on the subject of the shoulder.

The key to the soft tissue signs at the shoulders is the anatomy of the subacromial bursa and its extension, the subdeltoid bursa. This is the largest bursa in the upper limb, and for those interested in its anatomy and pathology Codman's text will be a delight.

RADIOLOGIC ANATOMY OF THE SUBDELTOID BURSA

The normal subacromial bursa can be demonstrated by percutaneous injection of a barium sulfate suspension at postmortem examination (15). The arm is to the side, ie, adducted, and the palm supine. The needle is introduced just lateral to the bicipital groove at the junction of the greater tuberosity and the humeral shaft. The postmortem bursagram shown in Fig. 2-1A and B was carried out with the needle tip just deep to deltoid and superior to the tuberosity.

The bursa cannot be defined in the soft tissues in the standard film of the normal shoulder joint, as it is a potential space only. The two layers of the extrasynovial fat bounding the bursa are in apposition (Fig. 2-2). However, the extrasyno-

Fig. 2-1. A subdeltoid bursagram carried out postmortem. Barium was used as a contrast agent and was injected by a scalp vein needle Anteroposterior (**A**) and inferosuperior (**B**) projections *(From Weston: Br J Radiol 42: 481, 1969.)*

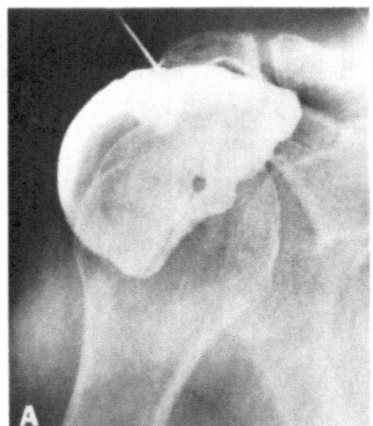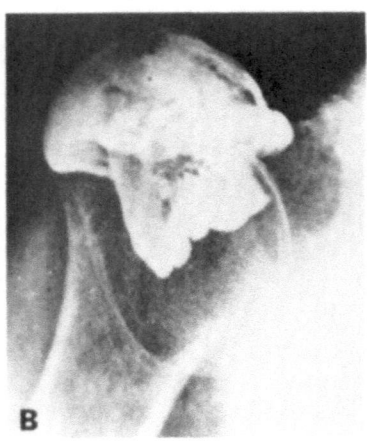

vial fat may be clearly defined on the plain anteroposterior film (with the humerus in external rotation) deep to deltoid and inferior to the acromion process and outer half-centimeter of the clavicle. This fatty layer runs along the outer margin of the upper end of the humerus for about 2.5 cm, and is 1 to 2 mm wide. It thus has the form of a thin crescent (Fig. 2-3). This crescent is often particularly well seen in the chest film of a child held up by the arms.

Soft Tissue Changes

In some patients the soft tissue outline of an enlarged subdeltoid bursa can be demonstrated in the plain anteroposterior film taken with the humerus in external rotation, because of its clear-cut outer, lower, and medial margin produced by the extrasynovial fat. The bursa has the shape of a teardrop. The enlarged bursa may act as a mass lesion and cause lateral displacement of the deltoid muscle (Fig. 2-4). Normally the deltoid outline is flattened at the level of the supraspinatus insertion. This segment, however, becomes convex in the presence of an enlarged bursa. These features can be appreciated by study of the line diagram of the case shown in Fig. 2-4A (Fig. 2-4B). The density of the deltoid muscle and subdeltoid bursa complex is increased (Figs. 2-5 and 2-6) (15). On occasion the extrasynovial fat of the bursa may not be seen caudally, only lateral displacement of the deltoid muscle being evident. This sign is combined with the increased density of the deltoid bursa complex. These features form the indirect signs of subdeltoid bursal enlargement. A distinction between direct and indirect evidence of subdeltoid bursa enlargement can thus be made, and should focus attention toward the shoulder joint as the possible site of the underlying lesion. Under some circumstances, either as a result of destruction by longstanding inflammatory disease or attrition of the rotator cuff, the head of the humerus is dis-

Fig. 2-2. Line diagram showing the extrasynovial fat about a normal subdeltoid bursa. The fat is shown by the cross-hatching and is a double layer of fat. *(From Weston: Br J Radiol 42:481, 1969.)*

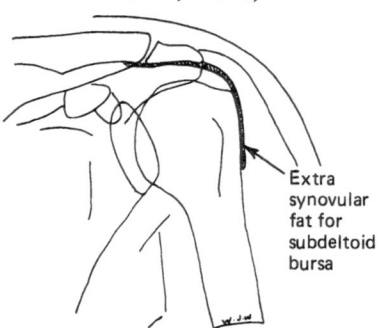

Extra synovular fat for subdeltoid bursa

Soft Tissues of the Extremities

Fig. 2-3. Normal extrasynovial fat about subdeltoid bursa (arrows). It is made up of two layers of fat as the bursa is a potential space only.

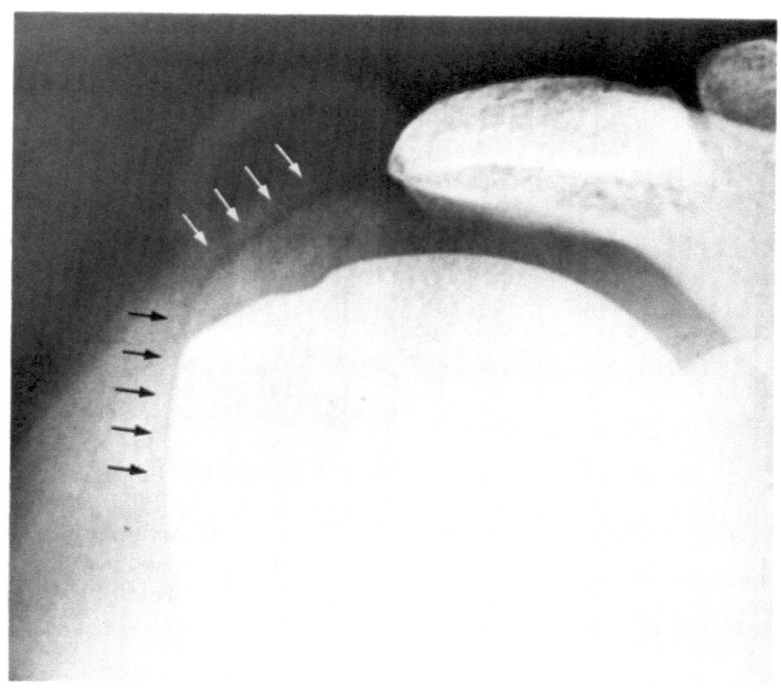

Fig. 2-4. **A.** Anteroposterior view of shoulder. Rheumatoid involvement of the enlarged subdeltoid bursa was well defined at the lateral, caudal, and medial margin by extrasynovial fat (arrows). It displaces the deltoid muscle laterally. (*From Weston: Br J Radiol 42:481, 1969.* **B.** Line diagram of **A.**)

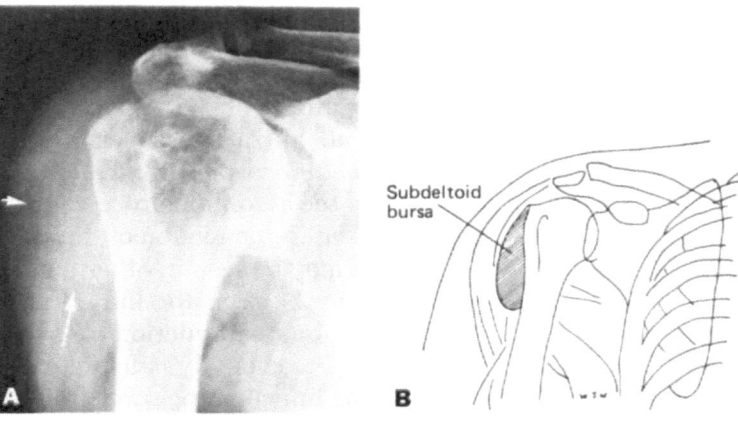

Fig. 2-5. Indirect evidence of enlarged subdeltoid bursa. The deltoid outline is rounded off by the enlarged bursa, acting as a mass lesion. Line diagram of abnormal right (**A**) and normal left (**B**) shoulders. The enlarged bursa is on the right side. (*From Weston: Br J Radiol 42:481, 1969.*)

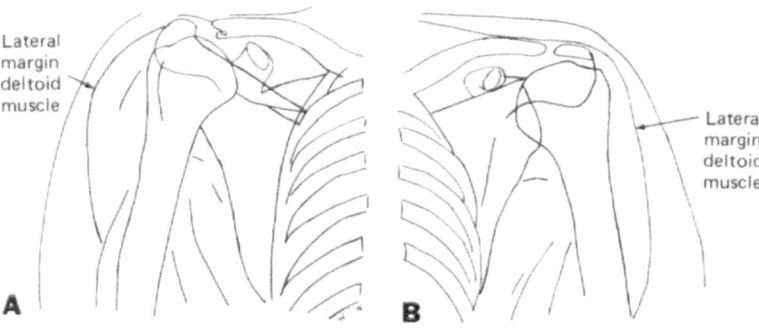

The Shoulder Region

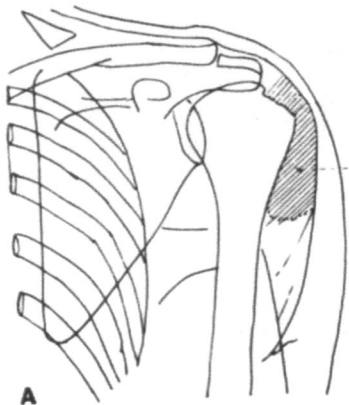
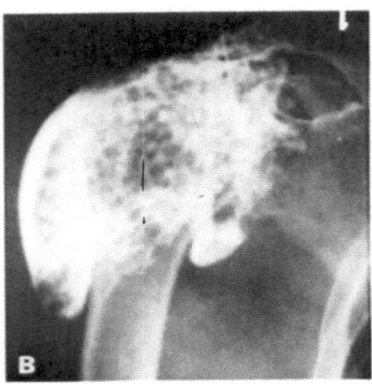

Fig. 2-6. **A.** Line diagram showing enlarged subdeltoid bursa producing a mass lesion with increase in density of deltoid muscle in that area. **B.** Arthrography showing subdeltoid bursal enlargement with nodular filling defects, typical of rheumatoid arthritis. (*From Weston: Br J Radiol 42:481, 1969.*)

placed upward beneath the coracoacromial arch by the unbalanced action of the deltoid muscle. The subacromial bursa is then obscured.

In the shoulder region dystrophic calcification is common. When present it serves as a natural guide to the radiologic anatomy of the region. The extrasynovial fat of the subdeltoid bursa lies superiorly, separating the tendon from the medial surface of the deltoid muscle and the inferior surface of the acromion process. Most commonly this calcification is seen in the tendon of the supraspinatus muscle (Fig. 2-7), but it may be seen in other tendons (Fig. 2-8). The calcified mass may be seen to shift in relation to other structures in the region on abduction of the shoulder.

Occasionally calcium salts may actually be found within the lumen of the subdeltoid bursa itself. Such a calcific mass is well defined, shaped like a teardrop, and extrasynovial fat may be seen over the lateral, caudal, and medial surfaces (Fig. 2-9).

Lewis (9) showed an area of calcification deep to the deltoid muscle (Fig. 2-10). It can be seen that this calcification acts as a mass lesion and displaces the deltoid laterally. Lewis considered that this lateral and downward extension of the calcific deposits, with a teardrop shape to its lowermost portion, was indicative of rupture into the surrounding soft tissues. In fact, this calcium would appear to be confined by the subdeltoid bursa.

Trauma may make evident various soft tissue structures. The radiolucency of extravasated fat is largely responsible for the various features which become apparent. Thus, recurrent dislocation of the shoulder may be associated with a li-

Fig. 2-7. Calcification in the tendon of supraspinatus.

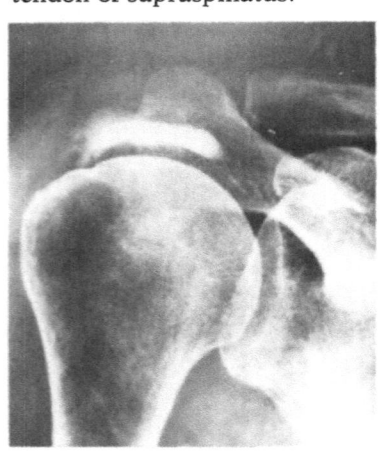

Soft Tissues of the Extremities

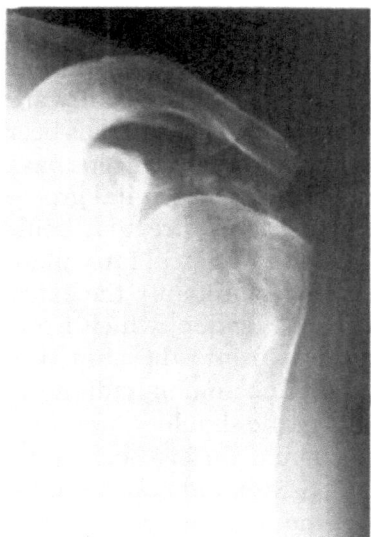

Fig. 2-8. Calcification in t
tendon of infraspinatus.

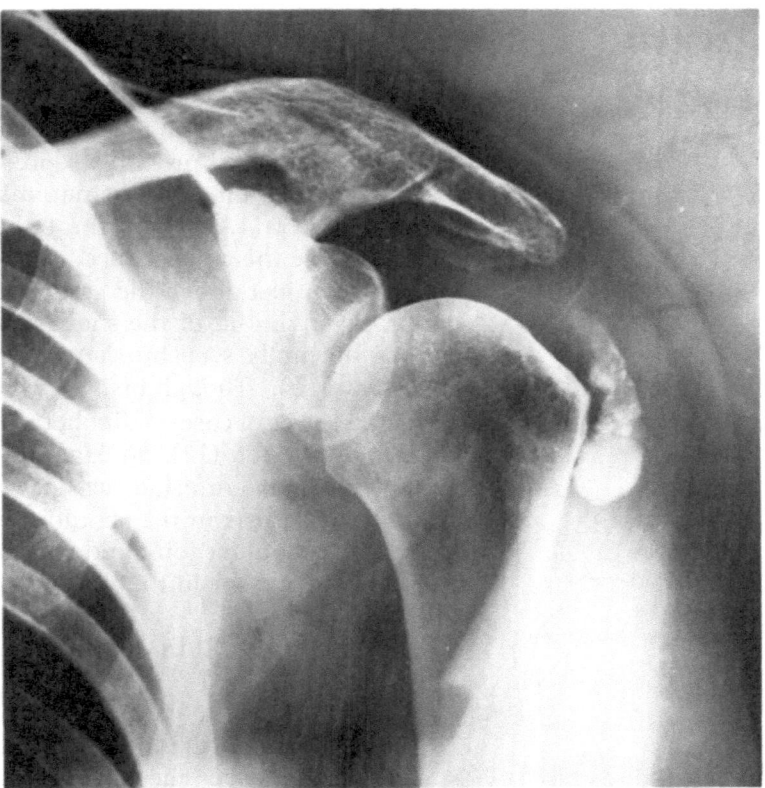

Fig. 2-9. A well-defined mass of calcium in the subdeltoid bursa, shaped like a teardrop. Extrasynovial fat is seen on its lateral, caudal, and medial surfaces.

Fig. 2-10. Calcification is noted deep to the deltoid muscle (arrow). (*From Lewis: The Joints of the Extremities, 1955. Courtesy of Thomas.*)

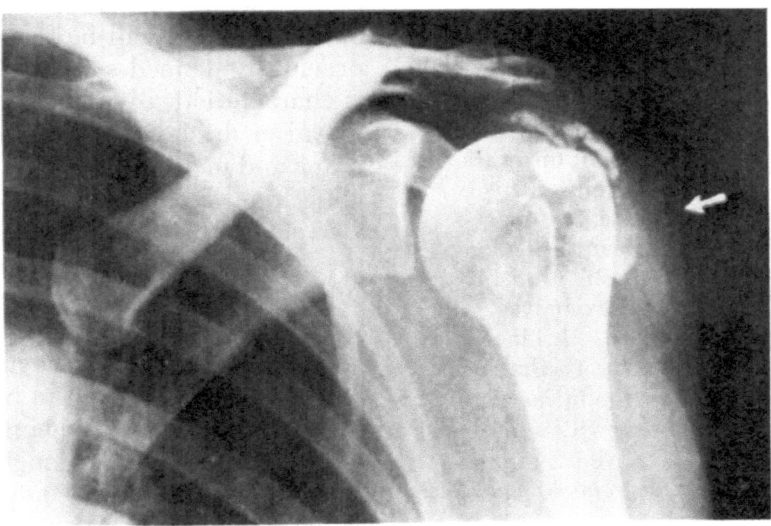

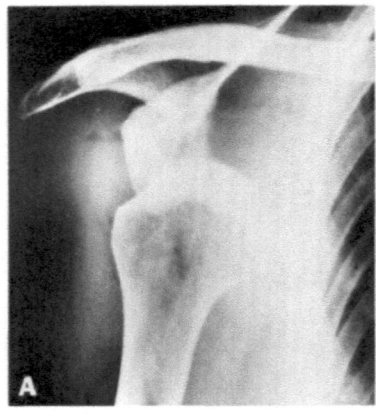

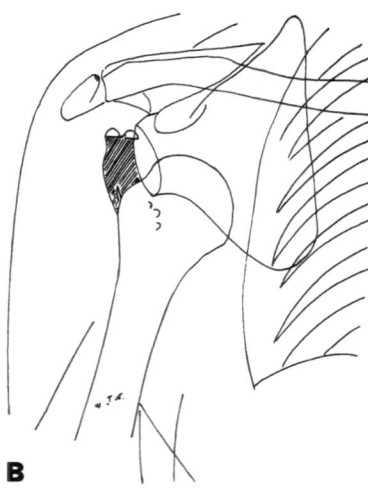

Fig. 2-11. A. An anterior subcoracoid dislocation of the shoulder is present. A fluid interface, separated into two halves, is seen within the capsule just lateral to the glenoid cavity. The appearances are those of a fat–blood interface as seen within an intact capsule in a case of recurrent dislocation of the shoulder joint. This is an erect film taken with a horizontal beam. The long head of biceps is probably the cause of the two halves to the fluid interface. **B.** Line diagram of **A.** The hatched area shows the intracapsular hemarthrosis with a fat–blood interface above it. (*From Weston: Australas Radiol 15:52, 1971.*)

Soft Tissues of the Extremities

pohemarthrosis of the joint visible in the erect film (18). The fat–blood interface opposite the glenoid divides the joint into two parts. A dome-shaped impression, convex caudally and extending down to the junction of the two interfaces, has been noted. This probably represents the long head of biceps passing down into the hematoma and on into the bicipital groove (Fig. 2-11A). It is the only anatomic structure that could cause this appearance. In Fig. 2-11A, the vertical fatty plane seen just above the greater tuberosity is probably the extrasynovial fat of the sheath about biceps tendon, which is not normally seen but here has been drawn into the joint (Fig. 2-11B). Though instructive this is an uncommon finding. In a series of cases of lipohemarthrosis of the shoulder presented by Saxton (12), no example of recurrent dislocation with a fat–blood interface was described. Saxton did note a lipohemarthrosis in the shoulder joint alone in some cases, and in the shoulder joint and subdeltoid bursa in others when a tear was present in the rotator cuff.

Rheumatoid Disease

Enlargement of the subdeltoid bursa is very commonly due to rheumatoid arthritis and may be the earliest manifestation of the disease. The enlarged bursa is usually evident on a plane film and acts as a mass lesion lying between the upper end of the humeral shaft medially and the deep surface of the deltoid laterally. The bursa has well-defined lateral, caudal, and medial margins because of its extrasynovial fat (Fig. 2-4), and is radiologically similar to an enlarged popliteal bursa where a well-defined superior margin is the diagnostic feature. The bursa may be outlined by a positive contrast study, either by direct injection of a contrast medium into the bursa itself or by contrast arthrography of the shoulder joint, as the bursa usually fills from the glenohumeral joint (14). The opacified bursa will be found to occupy the position of the previously defined soft tissue mass. The wall of the bursa is characteristically nodular and, occasionally, operative removal of the lesion allows the hypertrophic synovial membrane and melon-seed bodies responsible for this appearance to be seen. Such bursae may be huge, covering the deep surface of the entire deltoid muscle and extending up and over the shoulder joint beyond the normal medial limits of the subacromial bursa, to lie beneath the lateral insertion of trapezius and the lateral extremity of the clavicle (Fig. 2-12).

It is of interest that the articular surfaces of the shoulder have not been observed to be separated by fluid, even when involved by advanced rheumatoid changes. It is likely that any effusion escapes through an anatomic or pathologic defect in the rotator cuff (3).

In rheumatoid arthritis involving the shoulder joint (as has

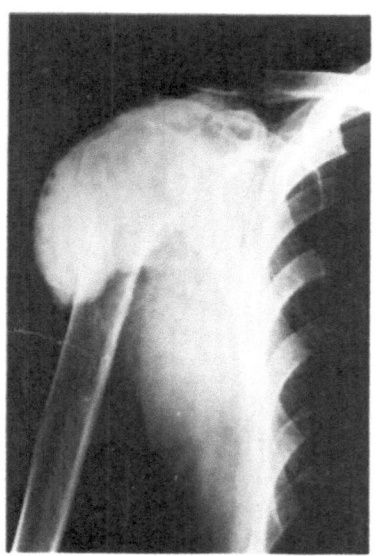

Fig. 2-12. Seropositive rheumatoid arthritis.
Arthrogram of right shoulder showing a large subdeltoid bursa. Note nodular filling defects resulting from localized synovial membrane thickening and melon-seed bodies. (*From Weston: Br J Radiol 42:481, 1969.*)

been noted in degenerative lesions of the rotator cuff) superior subluxation of the humeral head may occur, which obliterates the subacromial space and reflects wasting of the rotator cuff muscles with deltoid spasm or contracture.

RADIOLOGIC ANATOMY OF THE LONG HEAD OF BICEPS

The long head of biceps arises from the supraglenoid tuberosity at the upper margins of the glenoid cavity. It arches over the humeral head and passes through the bicipital groove where it has a synovial sheath (3). It has an elongated belly which can be separated anatomically from the belly of the short head to within 7.5 cm of the elbow joint.

Soft Tissue Changes

When the long head ruptures or separates from its origin the normal oval biceps belly separates into two obvious masses. One of these is the spherical belly of the short head of biceps, and the other is the elongated belly of the long head which is shaped like a stick of celery. As the long head is no longer under tension it moves distally, and becomes somewhat wavy in outline (16). Because of the anatomic arrangements of these bellies they are separated in this conditon right down to the region of the lower quarter of the humerus. At this point the two bellies fuse into a single mass which can be clearly seen in the radiographs (Fig. 2-13A and B).

Rupture of the long head of biceps is not an uncommon lesion, but the opportunity to carry out soft tissue studies is rather limited. Gilcreest (8) analyzed 100 such cases. X-ray examination was, however, usually stated to be negative. Arthrographic studies of the shoulder joint in this condition have been reported by Fischer (5) and by Ennevaara (4). The latter author, in his study of the painful shoulder in rheumatoid arthritis, found one case with rupture of the long head of biceps. He stated that de Seze (13) also had one case of rheumatoid arthritis in which there was a rupture of the biceps tendon. The authors have noted spontaneous rupture, presumably due to attrition, associated with severe secondary osteoarthrosis of the shoulder joint.

RADIOLOGIC ANATOMY OF THE SHOULDER JOINT

The articular surfaces of the shoulder joint are formed by the glenoid cavity of the scapula and the head of the humerus. The glenoid cavity is deepened by the labrum glenoidale, which is a circumferential rim of fibrocartilage. The cap-

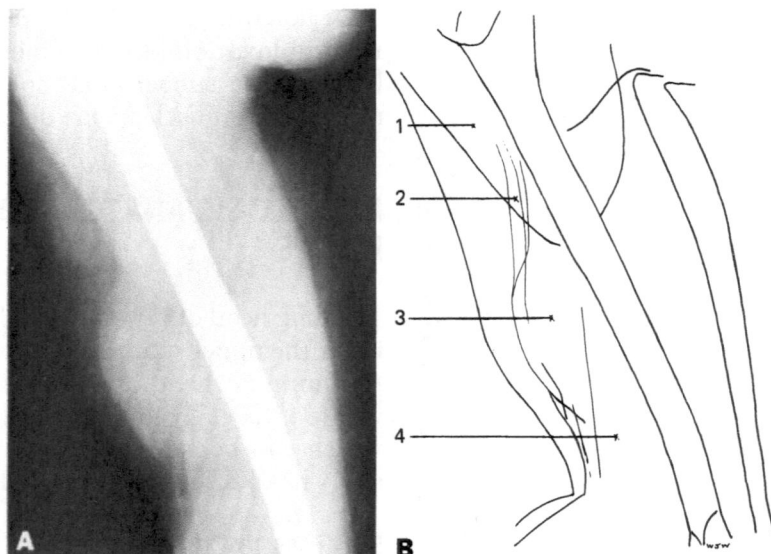

Fig. 2-13. A. Lateral view of the right upper arm demonstrates the soft tissue details accompanying rupture of the long head of biceps. The long head of biceps is seen as a thin wavy structure that unites with the main biceps mass just above the elbow area. **B.** Line diagram of **A,** showing the relationship of the short and long heads of biceps. The rounded belly of the short head of biceps is well demonstrated. 1, deltoid; 2, long head of biceps; 3, short head of biceps; 4, brachialis anticus. *(From Weston: Br J Radiol 42:539, 1969.)*

sular ligament is attached to the glenoid margin and the labrum glenoidale. On the humeral side it is attached to the edge of the articular cartilage above, but does extend out on to the shaft medially and below, the articular surface.

The capsular ligament is extensive and loose. When the muscles are cut from around the joint the humerus can be separated from the glenoid by an inch or more. This is the explanation for the observation that the humeral head can be depressed by a hemarthrosis of the glenohumeral joint and explains why the humerus may be elevated with rotator cuff degeneration.

There are two deficiencies in the capsule. The first is the foramen ovale through which synovial membrane becomes continuous with the large subscapular bursa, which lies between the neck of the scapula and subscapularis muscle. The second is opposite the upper end of the bicipital groove which is bridged by the transverse ligament. The tendon of the long head of biceps lies in this canal surrounded by a synovial sheath, continuous with the synovial membrane of the shoulder joint. Rarely, a defect in the capsule posteriorly allows the synovial membrane of the joint to become continuous with the bursa deep to the infraspinatus muscle.

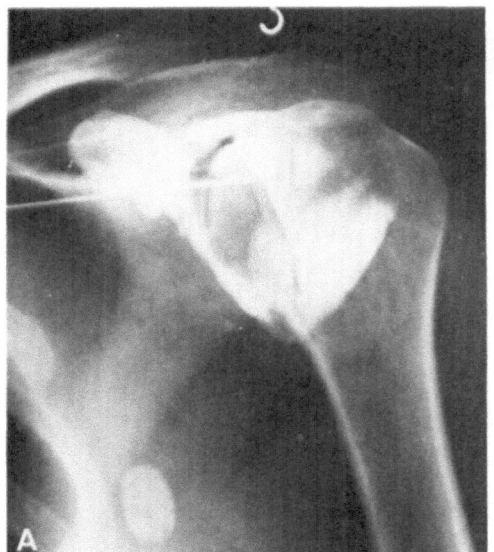 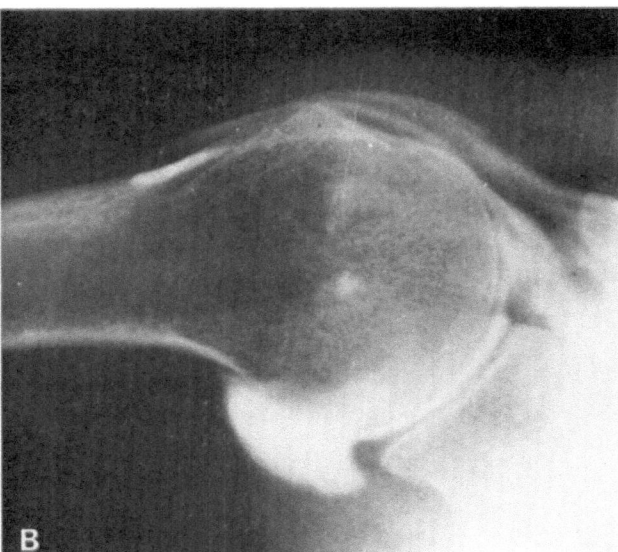

Fig. 2-14. A. Anteroposterior view of the filling phase of the normal shoulder joint arthrogram. **B.** Superoinferior view of the shoulder joint after instillation of 10 ml of contrast. The subscapularis bursa and long head of biceps are well shown.

The coracohumeral ligament runs from the root of the coracoid process to the greater tuberosity of the humerus. There are three glenohumeral ligaments thickening the deep surface of the joint capsule anteriorly. The superior one extends from the glenoid margin to the lesser tuberosity. The middle one runs below the foramen ovale to the lower part of the lesser tuberosity. The inferior ligament runs from the glenoid to the inferior aspect of the head of the humerus. Views of the normal arthrogram are shown in Fig. 2-14.

ENLARGED AXILLARY GLANDS IN RHEUMATOID ARTHRITIS

It was Ragan (11) who noted that generalized lymph node enlargement will appear in about one-half of patients with rheumatoid arthritis at some point in the course of the disease. A 67-year-old patient with seropositive rheumatoid arthritis presented with a rotator cuff lesion at each shoulder joint. On the plain film of the right shoulder the synovial reaction was noted in the subdeltoid bursa. Rupture of the rotator cuff was confirmed by arthrography. The villous hypertrophy of the synovial membrane and the joint mice could also be seen. Markedly enlarged lymph glands were noted in the axilla (17). They were demonstrated best on the radiographs taken on industrial film using the mammography technique (Fig. 2-15A–C). Contrast-filled lymphatic vessels,

The Shoulder Region

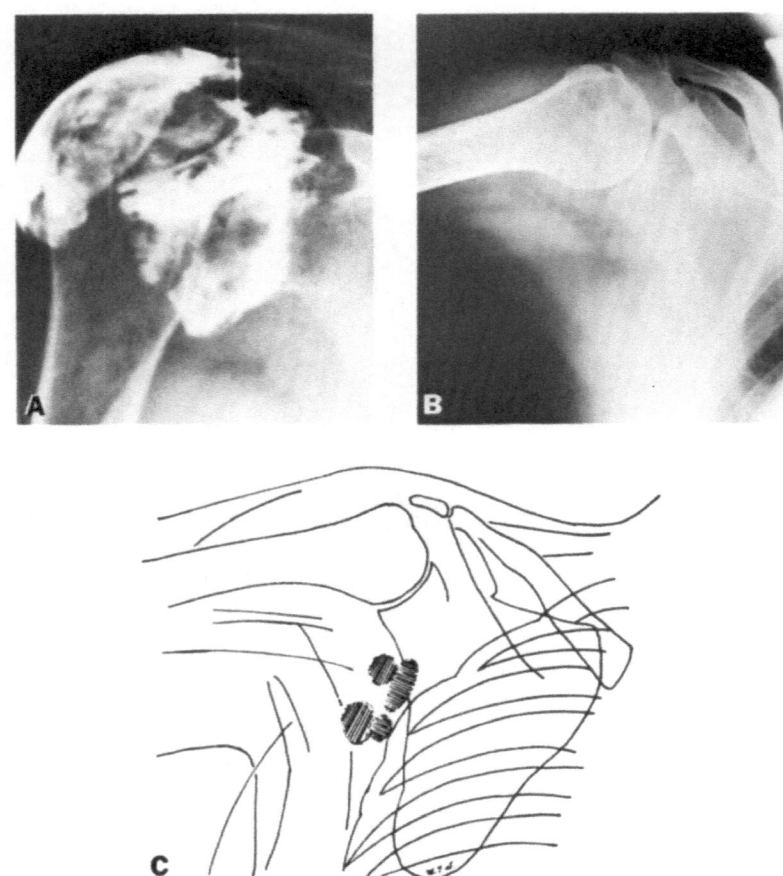

Fig. 2-15. **A.** Arthrogram with humerus abducted. The enlarged lymphatic glands are seen in the axilla. The subdeltoid bursa is filled by way of a tear in the rotator cuff. **B.** Enlarged glands demonstrated by mammography technique. **C.** Line diagram of **B.** (*From Weston: Australas Radiol 15:55, 1971.*)

Fig. 2-16. Arthrogram showing filling of subdeltoid bursa and glenohumeral joint. Contrast-filled lymphatic vessels are noted.

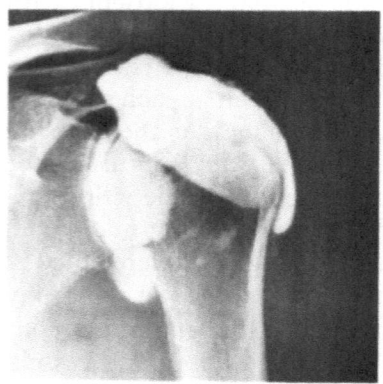

which we regard as a typical feature of the arthrogram in rheumatoid disease, were noted (Fig. 2-16).

INTRASYNOVIAL FATTY MASSES IN THE SUBDELTOID BURSA INVOLVED BY RHEUMATOID DISEASE

Translucent areas with a density of fat or lipid may be seen in synovial mass lesions in patients with chronic rheumatoid arthritis. Soft tissue masses were noted by Berens and Lin (2) to contain areas of translucency which in all probability represented large amounts of fatty material.

A patient with a 33-year history of seropositive rheumatoid arthritis presented with cartilage loss and erosions on the plain films. A large subdeltoid bursa was noted in which an

Soft Tissues of the Extremities

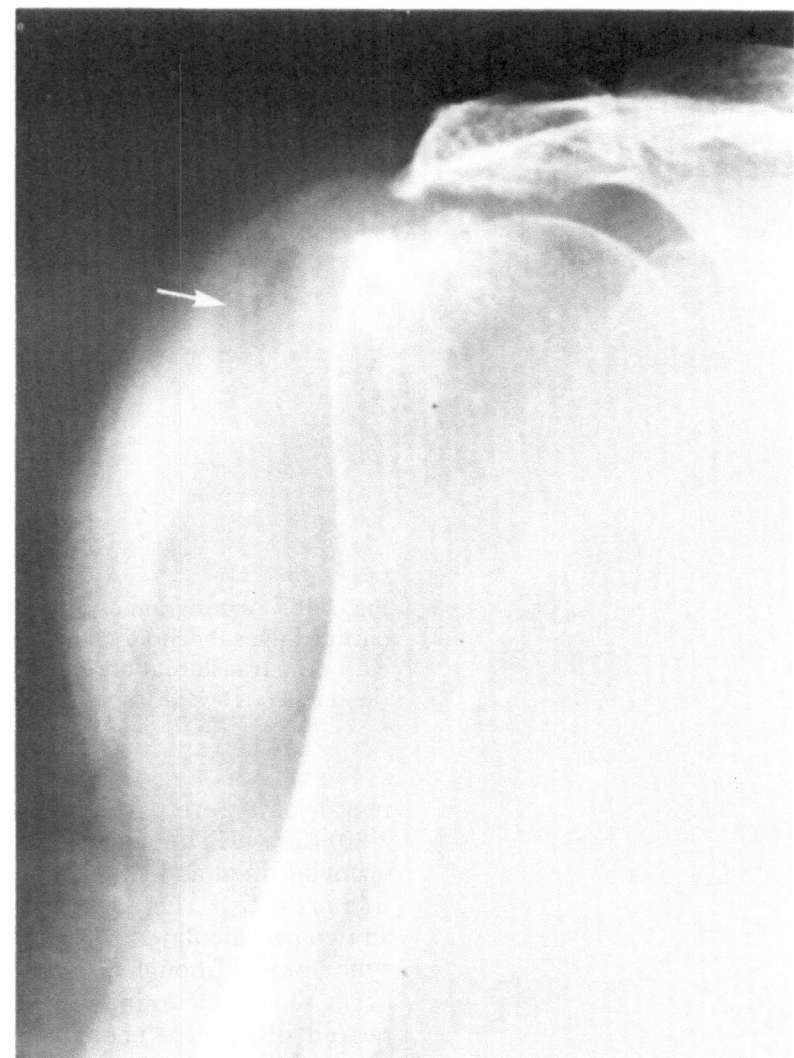

Fig. 2-17. Soft tissue anteroposterior view of right shoulder showing an enlarged subdeltoid bursa. An olive-sized translucent mass is noted deep to deltoid, having the density of fat (arrow). (*From Weston: Br J Radiol 46:213, 1973.*)

oval, translucent mass about 1.5 × 1 cm in area was present (Fig. 2-17). Arthrography of the glenohumeral joint was carried out. The contrast medium passed freely into the subdeltoid bursa indicating a rotator cuff defect. The glenohumeral joint cavity and the subdeltoid bursa were grossly enlarged. The translucent area was shown to be fixed to the lateral wall of the subdeltoid bursa and was clearly outlined by the contrast medium (Fig. 2-18). Many other filling defects were noted in both areas. At operation a lobulated fatty mass covered by synovial membrane was found on the lateral wall of the bursa (Fig. 2-19). Both the bursa and the glenohu-

The Shoulder Region

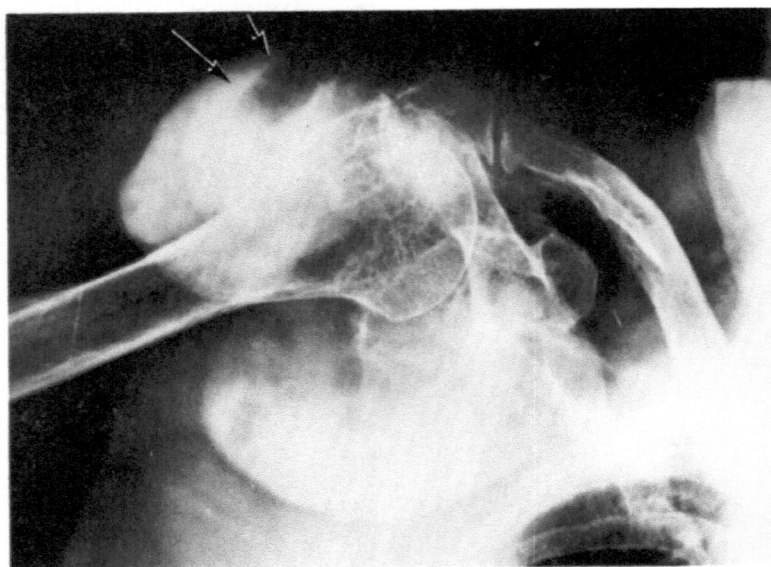

Fig. 2-18. Arthrogram of right shoulder. The opaque medium outlined the subdeltoid bursa, indicating a defect in the rotator cuff. The translucent area is clearly defined in the lateral wall of the bursa (arrows). *(From Weston: Br J Radiol 46:213, 1973.)*

meral joint were packed with large melon-seed bodies (Fig. 2-20) (20). Histologically the excised subdeltoid bursa was synovial-lined and showed changes consistent with rheumatoid arthritis. There was some fat present in its wall as well as two pedunculated lesions composed of fat and covered by synovium. Although fatty infiltration of synovial tissues may occur secondary to inflammation, these localized lesions appeared distinctive enough to justify the term "lipomata." The pedunculation and branching lobulation are further features characteristic of lipomata (10).

RADIOLOGIC ANATOMY OF THE ACROMIOCLAVICULAR JOINT

The trapezius muscle is inserted into the posterior border of the outer third of the clavicle, the inner border of the acromion process, and the upper lip of the posterior border of the spine of the scapula. The deltoid muscle arises from the corresponding outer margin of these three structures. The acromioclavicular joint is thus intimately related to the deep fascia and the overlying subcutaneous tissues. The joint has a capsular ligament thickened above and below by the superior and inferior ligaments. The superior acromioclavicular ligament is strengthened by aponeurotic fibers that extend between the trapezius and deltoid muscles (7).

Fig. 2-19. Soft tissue radiograph of the excised subdeltoid bursa with lobulated fat indicated by arrows. *(From Weston: Br J Radiol 46:213, 1973.)*

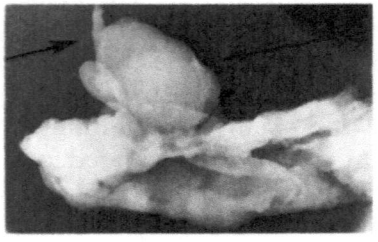

Soft Tissues of the Extremities

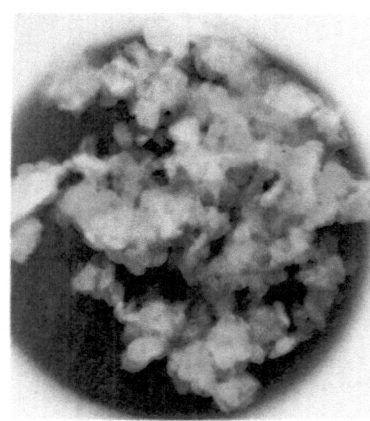

Fig. 2-20. Radiograph of melon-seed bodies that packed the bursa and the glenohumeral joint.

In many normal anteroposterior radiographs of the shoulder this aponeurosis on the superior aspect of the acromioclavicular joint linking the trapezius and deltoid muscles can be easily seen, provided the films are not overpenetrated (19). It dips after crossing the acromioclavicular joint, on the superior surface of the acromion, and continues up on to the origin of the deltoid muscle. It thus forms a shallow gutter over the acromion in the anteroposterior view.

Note is made of the arthrography of the acromioclavicular joint by Bateman (1). The surface marking of the joint corresponds to the prominent outer end of the clavicle. In most patients this outer end can be palpated, and arthrography is possible without television control.

Arthrography can be undertaken by puncturing the joint from its superior aspect. The needle (21-gauge butterfly) can be felt to pass through the superior ligament. One ml of contrast medium is sufficient to distend the joint and give adequate density. The joint cavity appears "L"-shaped and the horizontal limb of the joint passes under the outer end of the clavicle (Fig. 2-21) (21).

Soft Tissue Changes

Subluxation of the acromioclavicular joint produces three distinctive soft tissue signs (19).

1. Loss of parallelism of the extrasynovial fat of the subdeltoid bursa and the under surface of the outer end of the clavicle. When the acromioclavicular joint is subluxed or dislocated, a triangular gap may be seen between the under surface of the outer end of the clavicle and the extrasynovial fat of the subdeltoid bursa, which becomes continuous with the fatty plane on the superior aspect of supraspinatus muscle (Fig. 2-22A–C). Codman (3) noted that neither the subdeltoid bursa nor the supraspinatus

Fig. 2-21. Anteroposterior and inferosuperior views of the acromioclavicular joint: a postmortem examination. One ml of contrast medium has been placed in the joint. (*From Weston: Australas Radiol 18:213, 1974.*)

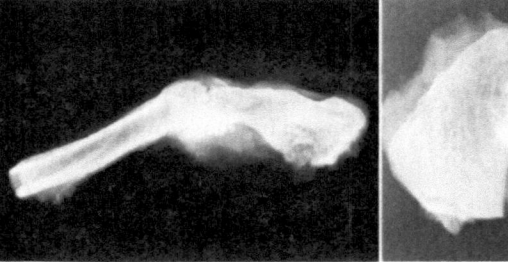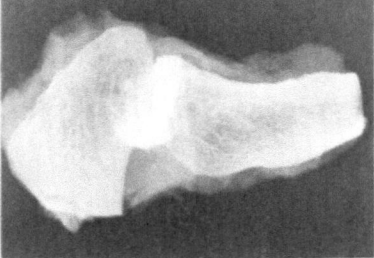

The Shoulder Region

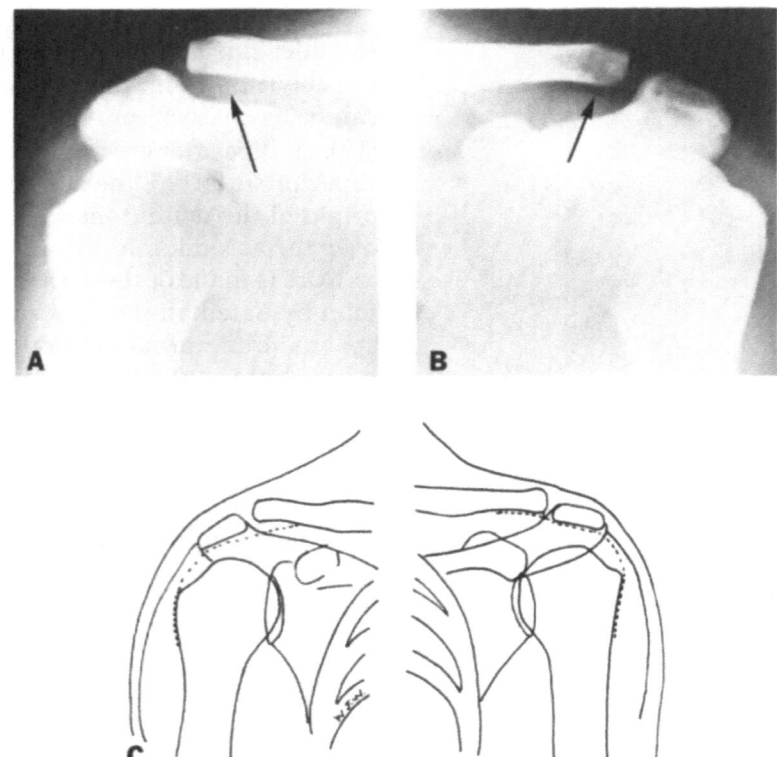

Fig. 2-22. A. Subluxation of the right acromioclavicular joint. The loss of parallelism between the extrasynovial fat (arrow) about the subdeltoid bursa and the under surface of the outer end of the clavicle is well demonstrated. **B.** The normal left acromioclavicular joint for comparison. Extrasynovial fat shown by arrows. **C.** Line diagram of **A** and **B**. The dotted line represents the two layers of extrasynovial fat of the subdeltoid bursa. (*From Weston: Br J Radiol 45:832, 1972*)

tendon are involved in acromioclavicular dislocation, as the bursa is attached to both the humerus and the supraspinatus tendon.

2. Soft tissue thickening deep to the aponeurosis on the superior aspect of the acromioclavicular joint and acromion process. The outer end of the clavicle and the acromion process are both vascular areas and, with trauma, edema and hematoma formation take place deep to the aponeurosis in this area. This exudate extends upward into the insertion of trapezius and separates the aponeurosis from the clavicle and the adjacent acromion. It produces a soft tissue mass over the cephalic aspect of the outer end of the clavicle and the acromion process, which can be clearly seen in all recent cases (Fig. 2-23). A striking change takes place in the region after 3 to 4 weeks. The soft tissue swelling settles, the outer end of the clavicle becomes un-

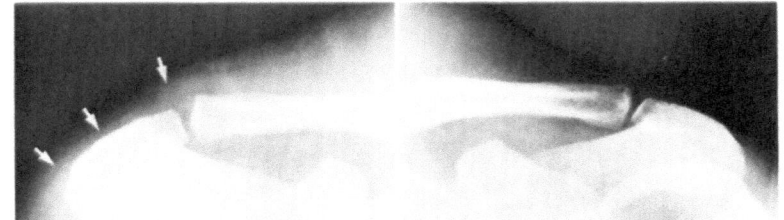

Fig. 2-23. A minor subluxation of the right acromioclavicular joint is noted. There is a mass lesion deep to the aponeurosis over the outer end of the clavicle and the upper surface of the acromion (arrows). The thickened origin of the right deltoid muscle is also visible. (*From Weston: Br J Radiol 45:832, 1972*)

duly prominent, and only then may the subluxation become apparent.

3. The beak-shaped origin of the deltoid muscle becomes "squared off" in the anteroposterior view. The superficial and deep surfaces of the deltoid muscle diverge at its origin from the acromion process, as seen in the anteroposterior view of the shoulder. The superficial surface of the muscle is outlined by the subcutaneous fat and the deep surface is demonstrated by the extrasynovial fat of the subdeltoid bursa. The exudate extends beneath the aponeurosis and on to the origin of deltoid muscle. This produces a "squaring off" of the beak-shaped origin of deltoid muscle, which can be seen in all recent cases with subluxation and dislocation (Fig. 2-23).

Good quality films are essential. With overpenetration these three signs are obscured. An anteroposterior view of both acromioclavicular joints must be taken as the soft tissue thickness varies from patient to patient. The loss of parallelism of the extrasynovial fat of the subdeltoid bursa beneath the under surface of the clavicle is the easiest sign to locate and the last to be obscured with overpenetration. These signs are particularly valuable in children where ossification of the clavicle is incomplete, and in patients examined supine where the subluxed joint may return to a near normal position. Under these circumstances the radiologist may be alerted by the soft tissue signs and this should lead to erect, weight-bearing views of the acromioclavicular joints.

Rheumatoid Disease

Involvement of the acromioclavicular joint by rheumatoid arthritis may be the principal cause of disability in the shoulder region. In addition to erosion of the articular surfaces, distension of the joint may lead to a soft tissue shadow which is best appreciated on the superior aspect of the joint

The Shoulder Region

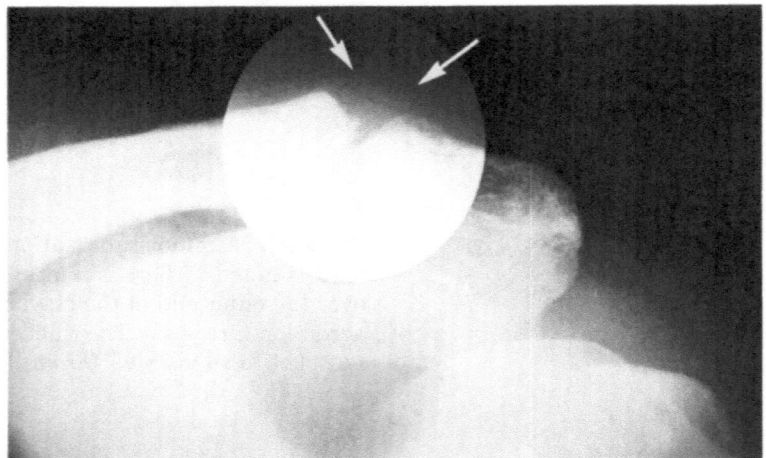

Fig. 2-24. Rheumatoid disease involving the acromioclavicular joint. A soft tissue swelling on the superior aspect of the joint is evident (arrows).

(Fig. 2-24). More advanced disease may lead to joint space widening from extensive erosion (osteolysis) and disruption of ligaments (Fig. 2-25).

RADIOLOGIC ANATOMY OF THE STERNOCLAVICULAR JOINT

The sternoclavicular joint is a double diarthrodial joint. The sternal end of the clavicle is larger than the articular facets on the manubrium sterni and the first costal cartilage.

Fig. 2-25. Advanced rheumatoid involvement of the acromioclavicular joint. "Osteolysis" of the bone ends.

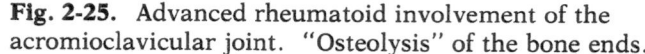

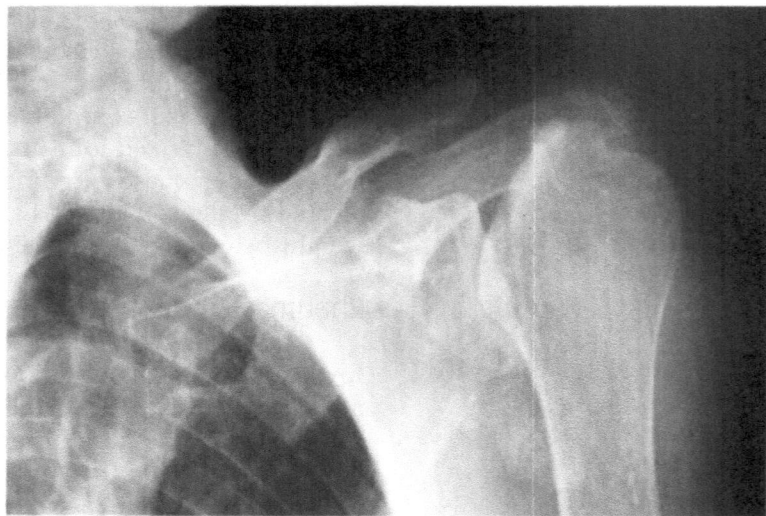

Soft Tissues of the Extremities

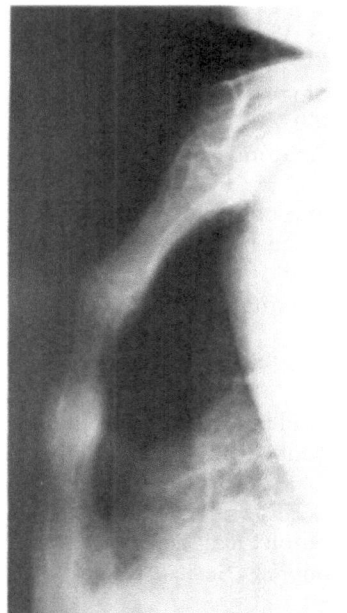

Fig. 2-26. Same case as in Figure 2-25. Forward subluxation of the medial end of the clavicle.

There is a capsule to the joint which is thin above and below, but is thickened by the anterior and posterior sternoclavicular ligaments. The anterior and posterior ligaments have fibers that pass down and in to the manubrium sterni. The interclavicular ligament runs from the upper and back aspect of the clavicle to the upper surface of the manubrium sterni. The rhomboid ligament is lateral to the joint and extends from the upper surface of the first costal cartilage to the rhomboid fossa on the under surface of the clavicle.

The articular disc is almost circular in outline and is thicker at the margin than in the center. It runs from the upper and back part of the clavicle to the inner end of the costal cartilage. It is attached to the joint capsule at its periphery and divides the joint into two parts.

Two synovial cavities are present, except when there is a small central foramen in the fibrocartilaginous disc.

Rheumatoid Disease

On occasion the sternoclavicular joint can be involved by the rheumatoid process. This leads to cartilage destruction and loss of bone from the inner end of the clavicle and from the articular surface on the manubrium sterni.

Lesions of the sternoclavicular joint are best demonstrated by posteroanterior tomography. Nevertheless, it is always worth having the standard posteroanterior views of the joints as the first step in the radiologic investigation. The loss of bone from the inner end of the clavicle and ligamentous disruption lead to joint space widening. This can proceed to forward subluxation, which can be demonstrated in a true lateral view of the sternoclavicular joint (Fig. 2-26).

Forrester and Nesson (6) state that "the changes of the clavicle do not occur in juvenile arthritis or ankylosing spondylitis; hence their appearance may be helpful in distinguishing rheumatoid arthritis from these two entities, since all three may cause identical changes in the cervical spine."

References

1. Bateman JE: The Shoulder and Neck. Philadelphia, Saunders, 1972, pp 134–137
2. Berens DL, Lin R: Roentgen Diagnosis of Rheumatoid Arthritis. Springfield, Ill, Thomas, 1969, p 180
3. Codman EA: The Shoulder. Rupture of the Supraspinatus Tendon and Other Lesions In or About the Subacromial Bursa. Brooklyn, Miller, 1934
4. Ennevaara K: Painful shoulder joint in rheumatoid arthritis. Acta Rheum Scand (Suppl) 11:1, 1967
5. Fischer FK: In Schinz HR, Baensch WE, Friedl E, et al (eds):

The Shoulder Region

Arthrography. Roentgen Diagnostics, Vol. 2. New York, Grune & Stratton, 1952, pp 1218–1277

6. Forrester DM, Nesson JW: The Radiology of Joint Disease. Philadelphia, Saunders, 1973, pp 383–389

7. Frazer JE: Buchanan's Manual of Anatomy, 6th ed. London, Balliere, 1937, pp 443–445

8. Gilcreest EL: The common syndrome of rupture, dislocation, and elongation of the long head of the biceps brachii. Surg Gynecol Obstet 58:322, 1934

9. Lewis RW: The Joints of the Extremities. Springfield, Ill, Thomas, 1955 p 9

10. Lichtenstien L: Bone Tumours, 2nd ed. St Louis, Mosby, 1959, pp 387–388

11. Ragan C: Clinical picture of rheumatoid arthritis. In Hollander JL (ed): Arthritis and Allied Conditions, 7th ed. Philadelphia, Lea & Febiger, 1966, pp 215–216

12. Saxton HM: Lipohaemarthrosis. Br J Radiol 35:122, 1962

13. de Seze S, Debeyre N, Manuel R: Radiological Aspects of Rheumatoid Arthritis. International Congress Series, No. 61 Amsterdam, Excerpta Medica, 1964

14. Weston WJ: Positive contrast arthrography in rheumatoid arthritis. Australas Radiol 12:141, 1968

15. Weston WJ: The enlarged subdeltoid bursa in rheumatoid arthritis. Br J Radiol 42:481, 1969

16. Weston WJ: The soft tissue signs with rupture of the long head of biceps. Br J Radiol 42:539, 1969

17. Weston WJ: Enlarged axillary glands in rheumatoid arthritis. Australas Radiol 15:55, 1971

18. Weston WJ: Recurrent dislocation of the shoulder with an intra-capsular lipohaemarthrosis. Australas Radiol 15:52, 1971

19. Weston WJ: Soft tissue signs in recent subluxation and dislocation of the acromio-clavicular joint. Br J Radiol 45:832, 1972

20. Weston WJ: The intrasynovial fatty masses in chronic rheumatoid arthritis. Br J Radiol 46:213, 1973

21. Weston WJ: Arthrography of the acromio-clavicular joint. Australas Radiol 18:213, 1974

Soft Tissues of the Extremities

CHAPTER 3

The Elbow Region

RADIOLOGIC ANATOMY

Bledsoe and Izenstark (2) observed that the anterior and posterior fat pads of the elbow joint are in fact extrasynovial, although intracapsular, and established the basis for the radiographic examination of the soft tissues at the joint.

The extrasynovial fat on the anterior aspect of the humerus is about 3 cm in length and 2 to 3 mm in width. In the lateral view of the elbow the fat runs from the joint line up along the ventral surface of the humerus. It can be seen on most radiographs and is only lost when there is gross overpenetration (Fig. 3-1A). On x-rays taken on industrial film it can be seen to continue downward to cross the joint line and to lie in close apposition with the radial head and neck (Fig. 3-1B). The posterior extrasynovial fat lies in the olecranon fossa and is thus not seen in the lateral view of the normal elbow joint. It is only when there is an effusion or synovial mass lesion in the joint that this fatty plane can be seen lying behind the humerus at the level of the olecranon fossa.

In the anteroposterior projection the extrasynovial fat, which can be seen to lie closely applied to the lateral aspect of the capitellum, crosses the joint line and continues downward over the lateral aspect of the head and neck of the radius. Lateral to the extrasynovial fat one can see the intermuscular fatty plane over the supinator muscle (Fig. 3-2).

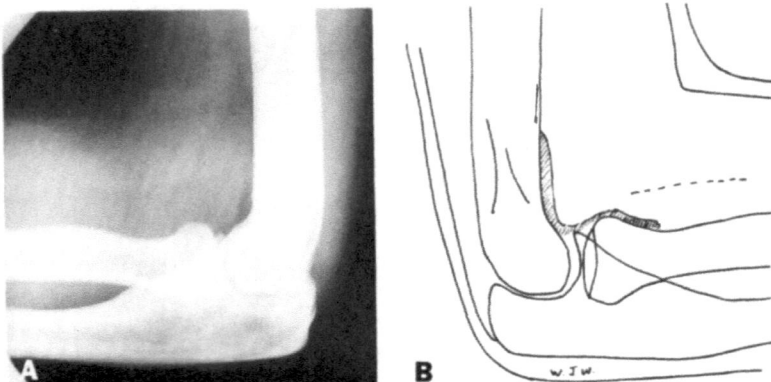

Fig. 3-1. **A.** Lateral view of a normal elbow joint. The extrasynovial fat lies anterior to the lower 3 cm of the humeral shaft and is 2 to 3 mm thick. **B.** Line diagram of lateral view of elbow. The hatched line represents the extrasynovial fat that extends down from the lower end of the humerus to cross the elbow joint and lie over the radial head and neck. It lies deep to the supinator fat line at the level of the neck of the radius.

Fig. 3-2. Line diagram of an anteroposterior view of a normal elbow joint, demonstrating the capsule of elbow joint where it is thickened by the annular ligament. 1, capsule of elbow joint thickened by annular ligament; 2, supinator fat line; 3, extracapsular fat. (*From Weston: Australas Radiol 15:170, 1971.*)

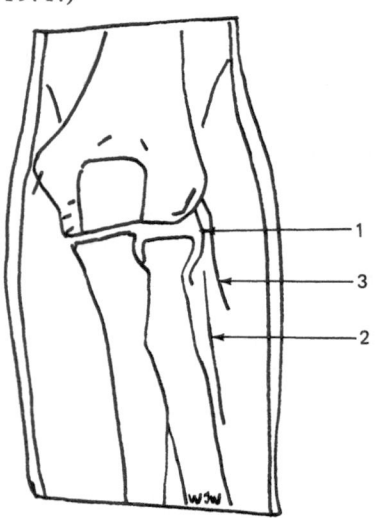

Rogers and MacEwan (11) described the normal fat plane overlying supinator muscle in the lateral view of the elbow joint. It can be seen as a line running parallel to the head, neck, and upper shaft of the radius. It is about 4 to 5 cm in length (Fig. 3-3). They reported that with traumatic effusions, synovial infections, and rheumatoid arthritis, not only were the synovial fat pads of the elbows involved but there was also a change in the fat plane overlying supinator muscle, in the lateral projection. This plane was displaced in the ventral direction.

Arthrography of the elbow joint can be carried out by injection from the lateral aspect between the radial head and capitellum. Four to 5 ml of contrast medium is sufficient to distend the joint.

A thin layer of contrast can be seen between the humerus, radius, and ulna in the anteroposterior view. There is a prolongation of the cavity distally that surrounds the head and neck of the radius. This is the membrana sacciformis as described by anatomists. The contrast extends up on the ventral aspect of the humerus for 3 cm and is shaped like the head of "Bugs Bunny," with two earlike projections (Fig. 3-4A). In the lateral projection the contrast can be seen to fill the olecranon fossa posteriorly, and it forms a convex-shaped mass anterior to the humerus. It extends down to and crosses the joint line and finishes with a linear-shaped mass deep to the fat plane over supinator muscle (Fig. 3-4B).

Soft Tissues of the Extremities

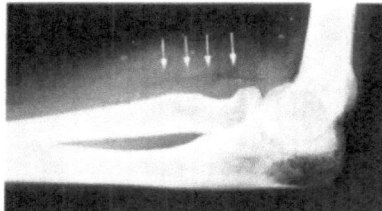

Fig. 3-3. Lateral view of elbow showing the supinator fat plane (arrows). It is about 4 to 5 cm in length and runs parallel with the head, neck, and upper shaft of the radius.

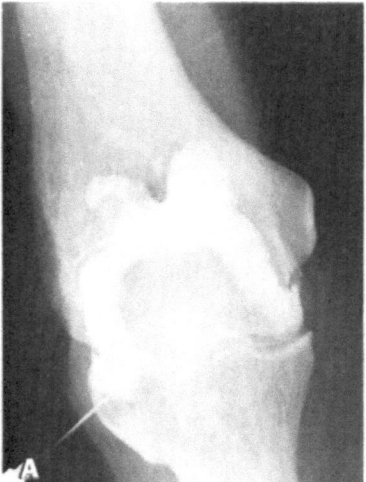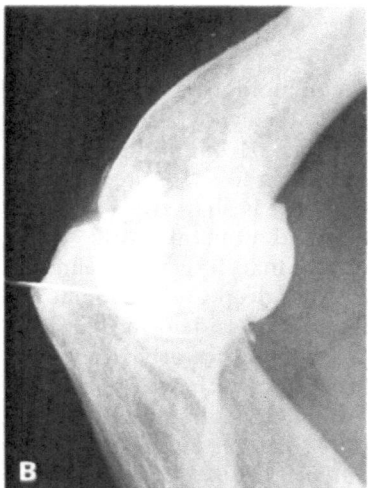

Fig. 3-4. **A.** Anteroposterior projection of normal arthrogram of elbow. Contrast extends up the humeral shaft for 3 cm and is shaped like the head of "Bugs Bunny." A thin layer of contrast extends into the joint space between the bone ends. The contrast has extended down and around the neck of the radius into the membrana sacciformis. **B.** Lateral projection of normal arthrogram. Contrast fills the olecranon fossa posteriorly. Anterior to humerus contrast is convex in shape. It extends down to cross the joint line as a thin strip over the neck of the radius. The membrana sacciformis is part of the synovial membrane of the elbow joint.

Fig. 3-5. Lateral view of elbow with large effusion. Dorsally extrasynovial fat is displaced out of the olecranon fossa and is convex posteriorly (arrow). Anteriorly the fat pad is shortened, thickened, and displaced ventrally. It becomes shaped like the left adrenal gland. Anteriorly two arrows show extrasynovial fat.

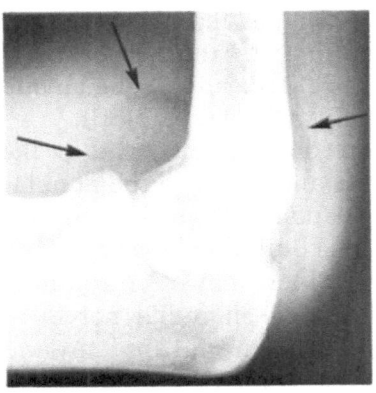

SOFT TISSUE CHANGES

Norell (8) noted that with traumatic effusions of the elbow joint there was displacement and deformity of the anterior and posterior fat pads. He termed these pads extracapsular, which was incorrect. As seen in the lateral view the extrasynovial fat plane is displaced ventrally away from the lower end of the humerus. The fatty plane is thickened and shortened and becomes shaped like the left adrenal gland as it sits on the corresponding kidney. Posteriorly the extrasynovial fat plane is displaced backward from the olecranon fossa and becomes visible as a fat pad convex posteriorly (Fig. 3-5). As the effusion is absorbed the extrasynovial fatty planes return to their normal position.

RHEUMATOID ARTHRITIS

Jackman and Pugh (5) noted that the synovial changes in rheumatoid arthritis were more prominent than those seen with trauma and infection. In rheumatoid arthritis one finds a synovial mass lesion which is due to effusion, synovial hy-

The Elbow Region

Fig. 3-6. **A.** Lateral view of elbow in patient with rheumatoid arthritis. Posteriorly the synovial mass lies between triceps and the olecranon fossa. Anteriorly the mass is shaped like a reversed numeral 3. Its caudal margin is well defined and lies deep to the supinator line, which is deformed and displaced anteriorly. They are outlined by extrasynovial fat. **B.** Line diagram of **A.** *(From Weston: Australas Radiol 15:170, 1971.)*

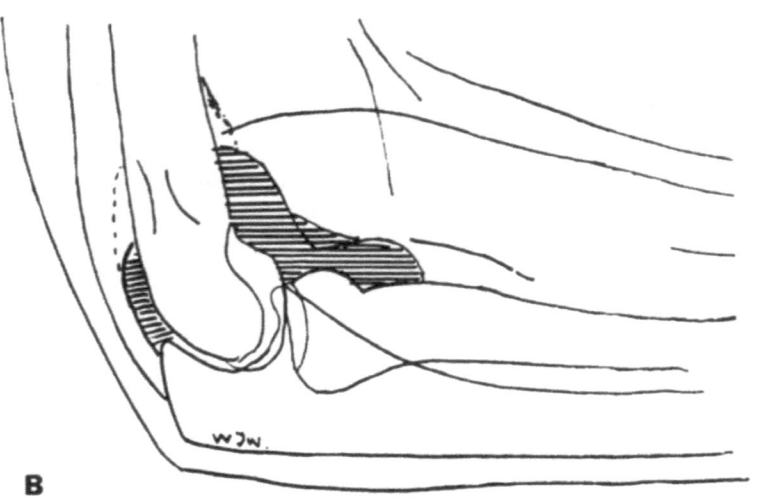

Fig. 3-7. Line diagram of sagittal section of the elbow joint. The synovial cavity is in the cross-hatched area. 1, triceps muscle; 2, extensor carpi ulnaris muscle; 3, radial nerve; 4, brachialis muscle; 5, brachioradialis muscle; 6, extensor carpi radialis longus muscle; 7, deep radial nerve (posterior interosseous nerve); 8, supinator line; 9, supinator muscle. *(After von Lanz and Wachsmuth: Praktische Anatomie, Springer-Verlag, 1959.)*

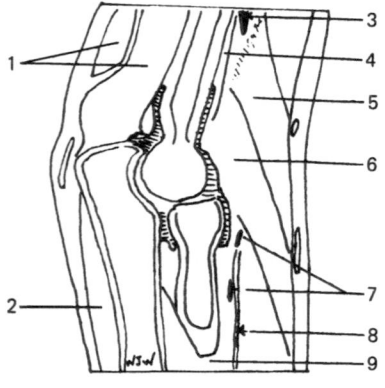

pertrophy, joint mice, and edema. The synovial changes take on a pattern which is predictable unless sacculation has occurred (3,9). Saccules vary in size from case to case.

In the lateral view the synovial mass posteriorly is noted to lie between triceps and the olecranon fossa of the humerus. Anteriorly the pattern is seen to be shaped like a reversed numeral 3 (Fig. 3-6A) where it is outlined by the extrasynovial fat. This pattern has been described in part by Jackman and Pugh (5) and by Rogers and MacEwan (11) (Fig. 3-6B).

The supinator fat line is involved and is distorted by the synovial mass that lies beneath it and distal to the annular ligament that is disrupted. Its caudal margin is well outlined by the extrasynovial fat and is bull-nosed in shape (16). This involvement also explains why there may be entrapment of the posterior interosseous nerve (deep radial nerve) in some of these patients (7). The normal synovial anatomy and its relationship with the deep radial nerve (13) are shown in the sagittal section of the elbow joint (Fig. 3-7).

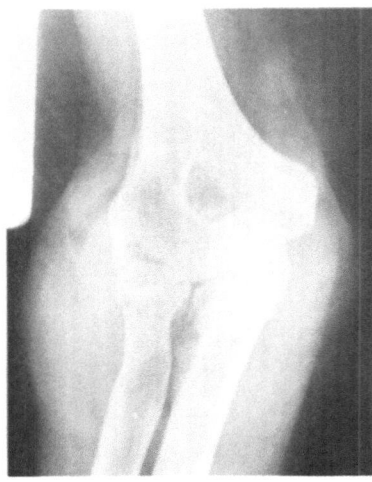

Fig. 3-8. Anteroposterior view of elbow in patient with rheumatoid arthritis. The dense mass lesion lies lateral to the capitellum and head and neck of radius, and displaces the joint capsule laterally. (*From Weston: Australas Radiol 15:170, 1971.*)

In the anteroposterior projection, the synovial mass lesion can be seen lateral to the joint space and to the head and neck of the radius (Fig. 3-8). This mass lesion causes capsular displacement as well as an increase in density. It is easily demonstrated when contrast arthrography is performed (Figs. 3-9A and B, 3-10A and B) and produces the displacement of the supinator line as seen in the lateral view. A further mass lesion can be seen on the medial aspect of the joint line when adequate soft tissue detail has been obtained. It can thus be understood why the ulnar nerve may be involved in this area when pressed on by the synovial mass (Fig. 3-11).

The arthrographic findings in rheumatoid arthritis are similar to those seen in the shoulder. Both the synovial hypertrophy and possible fibrin bodies contribute to the appearances. In one case the contrast outlined the lymphatics and the supratrochlear glands (6,14). The authors feel this appearance is specific to rheumatoid arthritis, although Staple (12) states he has seen this appearance following trauma (Fig. 3-12).

Ball (1) stated that "I think that one sometimes sees lymphatics literally stuffed with lymphocytes in rheumatoid synovia, which would suggest to me that there may, indeed, be some circulation from the locus to the neighboring lymph nodes."

Sacculation of the joint capsule at the elbow, more particularly on the medial and lateral aspects, is common. On the lateral aspect a cystic swelling may protrude between the an-

Fig. 3-9. A. Lateral view of arthrogram in Still's disease. The synovial membrane is hypertrophic and nodular. The distal portion displaces the supinator line ventrally. **B.** Anteroposterior view showing a synovial mass on the lateral aspect of the elbow joint. (*From Weston: Australas Radiol 15:170, 1971.*)

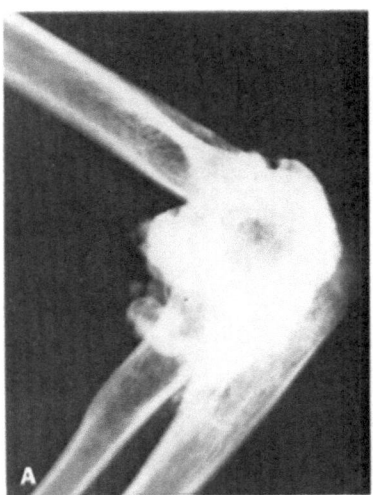
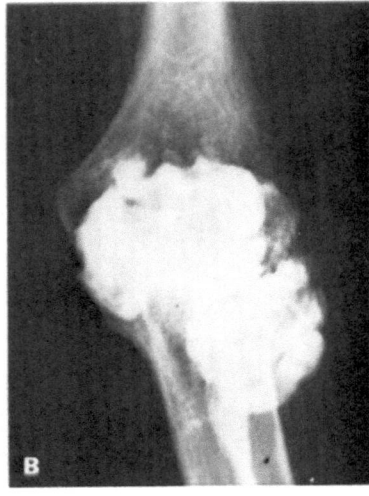

The Elbow Region

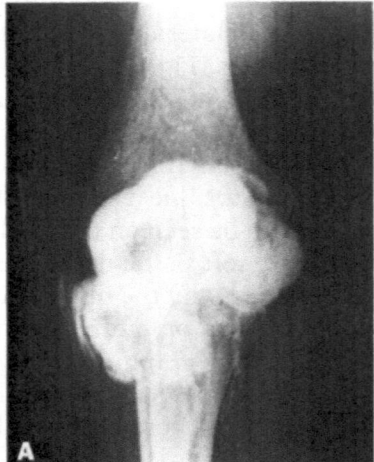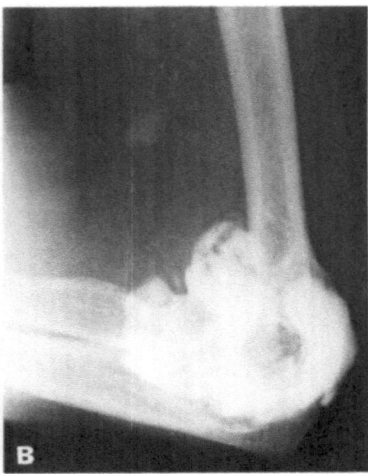

Fig. 3-10. A. Anteroposterior view of arthrogram in patient with active rheumatoid arthritis. A synovial mass extends from the lateral aspect of the joint line. Minor extravasation of contrast material through the puncture track on the lateral aspect. Lymphatic filling is noted on the medial side of the joint. **B.** Lateral view. The synovial mass is shaped like a reversed numeral 3 (synovial bird). Lymphatic vessels and supratrochlear lymph nodes are filled as well. (*From Weston: Australas Radiol 15:170, 1971.*)

terior and posterior bands of the lateral ligament, or there may be an hourglass swelling with an additional protrusion behind the posterior band (Fig. 3-13).

Rupture of the rheumatoid elbow is uncommon (4), but its occurrence illustrates a further parallel between the antecubital fossa and posterior sacculation at the knee. Figure 3-14

Fig. 3-11. Anteroposterior view of elbow of patient with rheumatoid arthritis. A mass lesion can be seen on the medial and lateral aspects of the joint line.

Fig. 3-12. Lateral radiograph of the left elbow. A large synovial mass is noted anteriorly which displaces the supinator line. Rounded translucent areas of fat are seen within the mass. **B.** Line diagram of **A.** (*From Weston: Br J Radiol 46:213, 1973.*) (18)

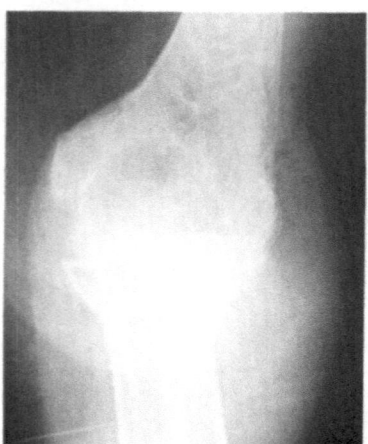

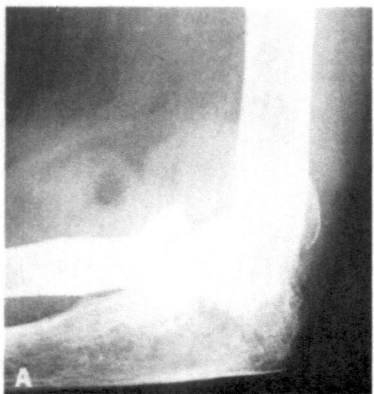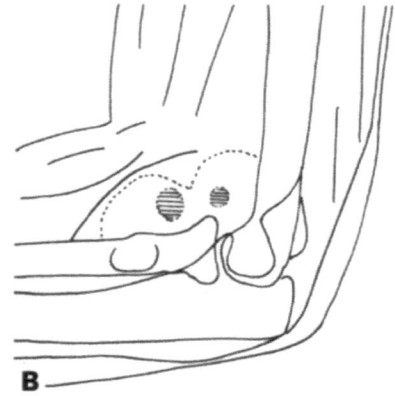

Soft Tissues of the Extremities

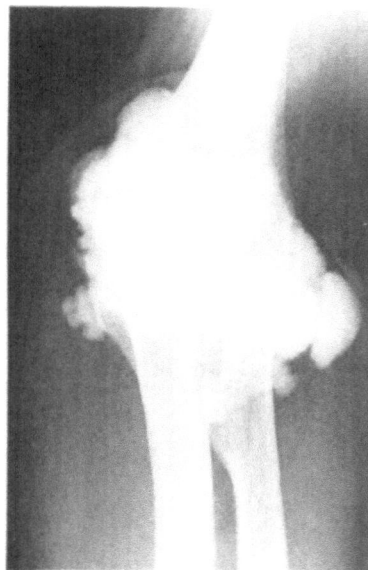

Fig. 3-13. Anteroposterior view of arthrogram in a rheumatoid patient. Sacculation of the joint capsule is shown on the lateral aspect of the joint.

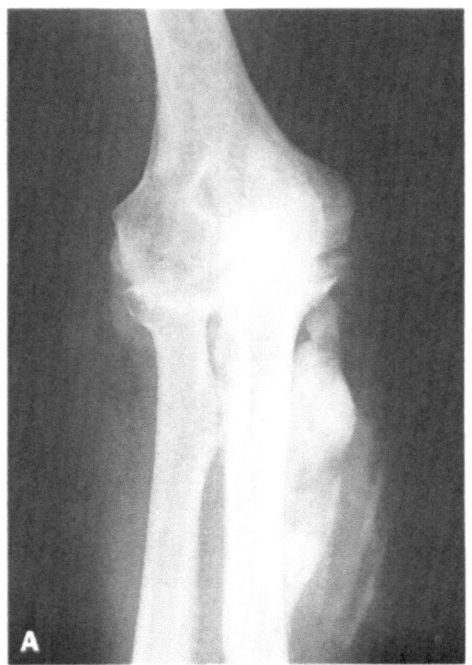

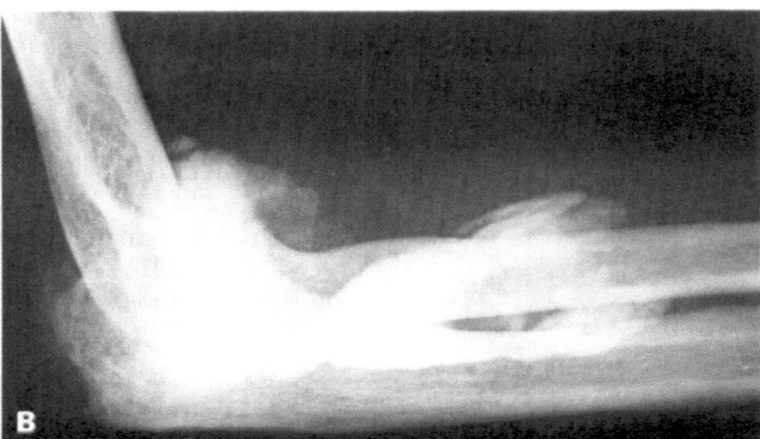

Fig. 3-14. An arthrogram of the elbow in a patient with rheumatoid arthritis. There has been sacculation and then rupture. **A.** Anteroposterior view. **B.** Lateral view with irregular outline of contrast in mid forearm indicating rupture.

illustrates rupture of the elbow joint in a patient who also later developed an extensive multiloculated cyst in the calf.

THE SUPRATROCHLEAR GLANDS

Enlarged supratrochlear glands can be seen in the soft tissues in patients with rheumatoid arthritis of the elbow. One, two, or three glands have been noted in the soft tissues in this type

The Elbow Region

Fig. 3-15. A long synovial-lined cavity on dorsum of ulna. This most probably resulted from sacculation of the olecranon bursa. (*Professor K. Vainio, Finland*)

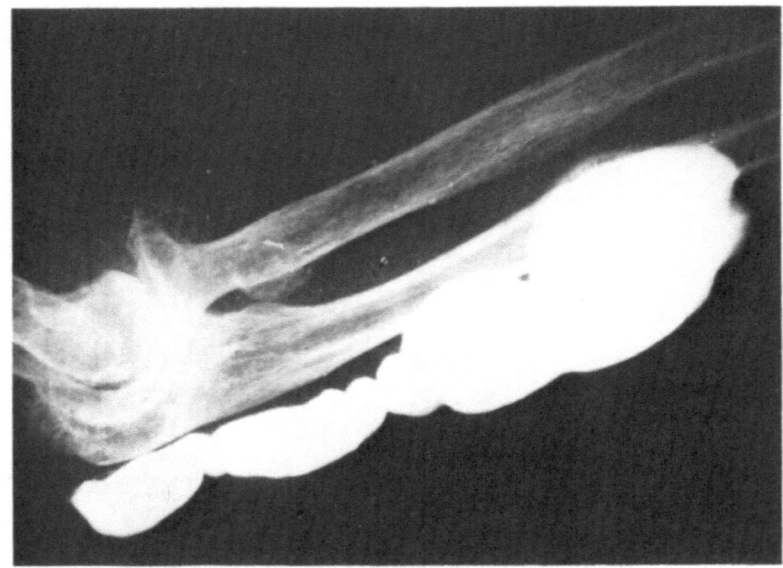

of case (17). Ragan (10) has discussed the problem of lymphatic enlargement in rheumatoid arthritis (Fig. 3-15).

THE OLECRANON BURSA AND SUBCUTANEOUS NODULES

The normal olecranon bursa lies like a cap over the olecranon process (Fig. 3-16). It can be outlined easily by contrast material percutaneously (15).

Fig. 3-16. Lateral view of the normal olecranon bursa outlined by barium at postmortem examination. An arthrogram has also been peformed on the elbow joint. (*From Weston: Australas Radiol 14:323, 1970.*)

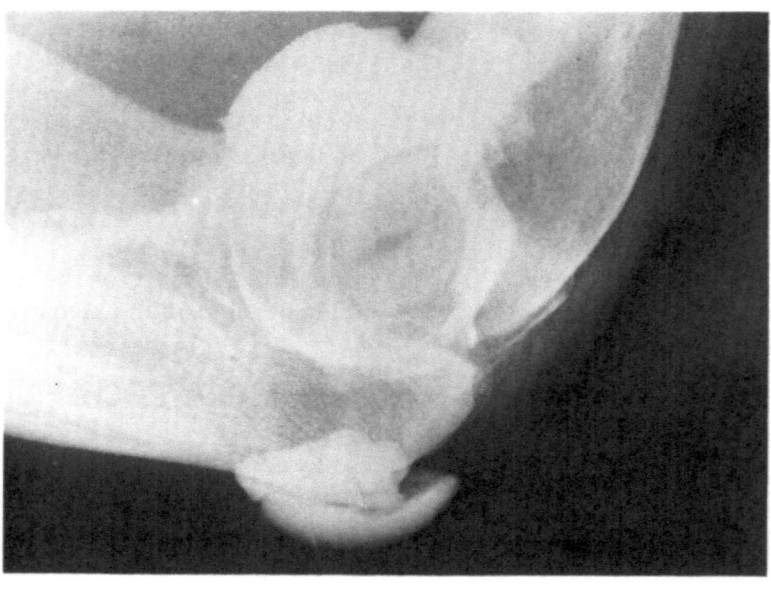

Soft Tissues of the Extremities

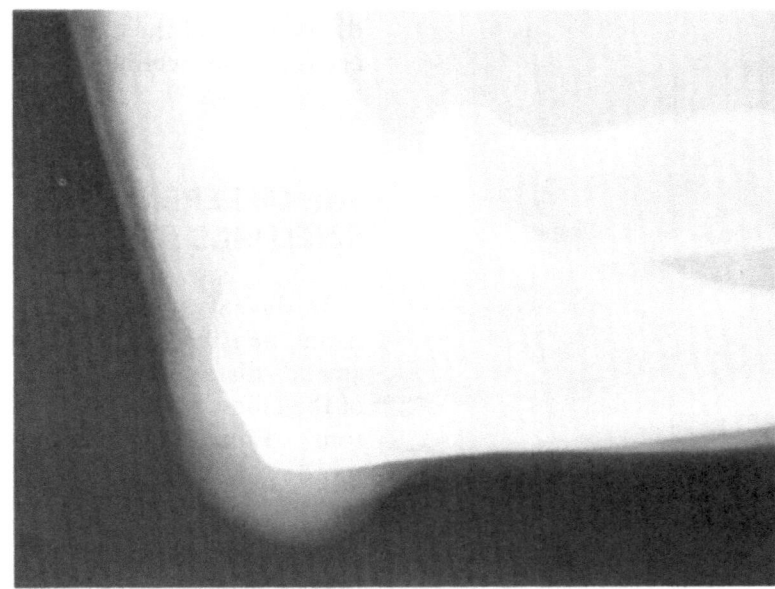

Fig. 3-17. The olecranon bursa is distended by an effusion and is homogeneous in density.

On the extensor aspect of the ulna just below the elbow, both distension of the olecranon bursa (Fig. 3-17) and the development of subcutaneous rheumatoid nodules (Fig. 3-18) may produce soft tissue swelling. On occasion the olecranon bursa may be markedly distended with saccular protrusion extending down the dorsal aspect of the forearm. Patients thus affected may even experience paresthesias within the

Fig. 3-18. Rheumatoid nodules at the posterior aspect of the upper end of the ulna. The reticular pattern of connective tissue strands distinguishes these nodules from an effusion into the olecranon bursa.

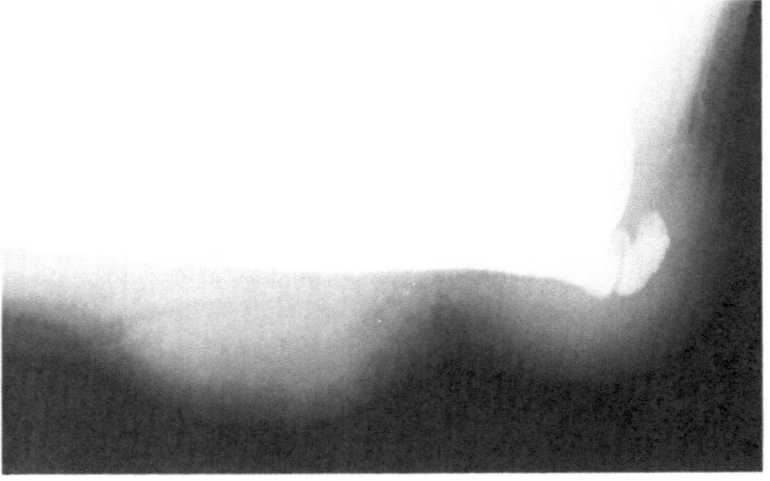

The Elbow Region

distribution of the ulnar nerve when moderate pressure is exerted on the swelling.

THE DIFFERENTIATION OF LOCALIZED SWELLINGS AT THE ELBOW

In the soft tissue x-ray a distended bursa is of a homogeneous density, but a reticular pattern of connective tissue strands distinguishes a nodule. In oblique views sacculation of the elbow may produce localized swellings of similar contour. Enlarged supratrochlear nodes are situated rather more proximally.

References

1. Ball J: Early Synovectomy in Rheumatoid Arthritis. Amsterdam, Excerpta Medica, 1964, p 22
2. Bledsoe RC, Izenstark JL: Displacement of fat pads in disease and injury of the elbow. A new radiographic sign. Radiology 73:717, 1959
3. Ehrlich GE: Antecubital cysts in rheumatoid arthritis. A corollary to popliteal (Baker's) cyst. J Bone Joint Surg [Am] 54:165, 1972
4. Goode JD: Synovial rupture of the elbow joint. Ann Rheum Dis 27:604, 1968
5. Jackman RJ, Pugh DG: The positive elbow fat pad sign in rheumatoid arthritis. Am J Roentgenol 108:812, 1970
6. Lewin JR, Mulhern LM: Lymphatic visualization during contrast arthrography of the knee. Radiology 103:577, 1972
7. Marmor L, Lawrence JF, Dubois EL: Posterior interosseous nerve palsy due to rheumatoid arthritis. J Bone Joint Surg [Am] 49:381, 1967
8. Norell HG: Roentgenologic visualisation of the extracapsular fat. Its importance in the diagnosis of traumatic injuries to the elbow. Acta Radiol (Stockh) 42:205, 1954
9. Palmer DG: Synovial cysts in rheumatoid disease. Ann Intern Med 70:61, 1969
10. Ragan C: Arthritis and allied conditions. In Hollander JL (ed): A Textbook of Rheumatology, 7th ed. 1966, pp 215–216
11. Rogers SL, MacEwan DW: Changes due to trauma in the fat plane overlying the supinator muscle. A radiological sign. Radiology 92:954, 1969
12. Staple TW: Personal communication, 1972
13. von Lanz T, Wachsmuth W: Praktische Anatomie, Erster Band Brittereil, Arm. Vol. 2. Berlin, Springer-Verlag, 1959
14. Weston WJ: Lymphatic filling during positive contrast arthrography in rheumatoid arthritis. Australas Radiol 13:368, 1969

15. Weston WJ: The olecranon bursa. Australas Radiol 14:323, 1970
16. Weston WJ: The synovial changes at the elbow in rheumatoid arthritis. Australas Radiol 15:170, 1971
17. Weston WJ: Enlarged supratrochlear lymphatic glands in rheumatoid arthritis. Australas Radiol 12:260, 1968
18. Weston WJ: The intrasynovial fatty masses in chronic rheumatoid arthritis. Br J Radiol 46:213, 1972

CHAPTER 4

The Wrist and Hand

Resnick (28) has written an excellent paper, which should be read by all those interested in the anatomy of the wrist.

The prestyloid recess of the radiocarpal joint is normally in intimate contact with the ulnar styloid process (Fig. 4-1A). The pisicuneiform joint has a separate synovial cavity under these conditions. However, in 34 percent (15,16) of cases the radiocarpal joint communicates with the pisicuneiform joint (Fig. 4-1B). The tendon of extensor carpi ulnaris is related to the posterior aspect of the head of the ulna and to the ulnar styloid process (Fig. 4-1C). These three synovial structures are commonly involved in rheumatoid arthritis and lead to the synovial mass lesions seen on the medial aspect of the wrist.

There is a variable relationship between the deep fascia, the tip of the ulnar styloid process, and the medial aspect of the carpus. The line of the deep fascia follows the configuration of the fascia–fat interface in the soft tissue radiograph. In some cases this line runs parallel to the ulnar styloid process; but in others it diverges from it as the line passes toward the carpus (Fig. 4-2). There does not appear to be any association between the length of the ulnar styloid process and the particular form of the fascia–fat interface in this area. The relationship of the synovial membrane at the wrist to the deep fascia in the region of the ulnar styloid process explains why the soft tissue changes in this area are well seen. The great bulk of the synovial membrane, ie, radiocarpal joint, pi-

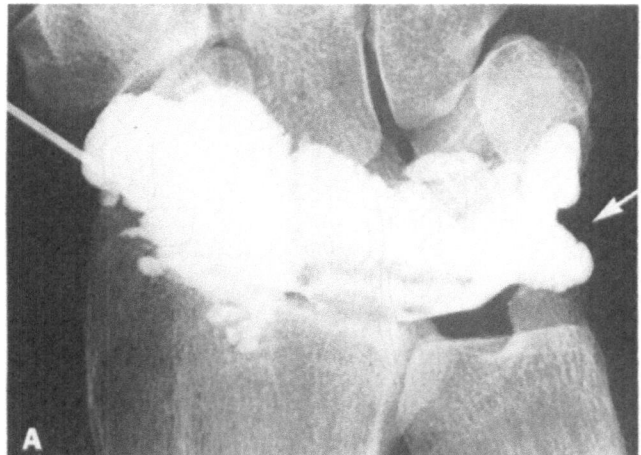

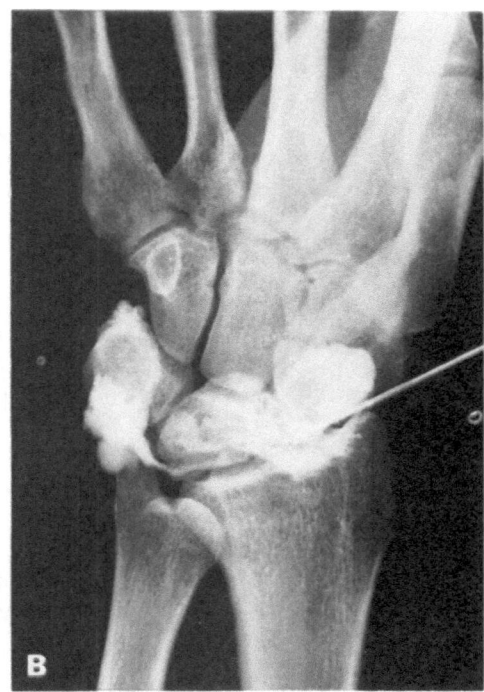

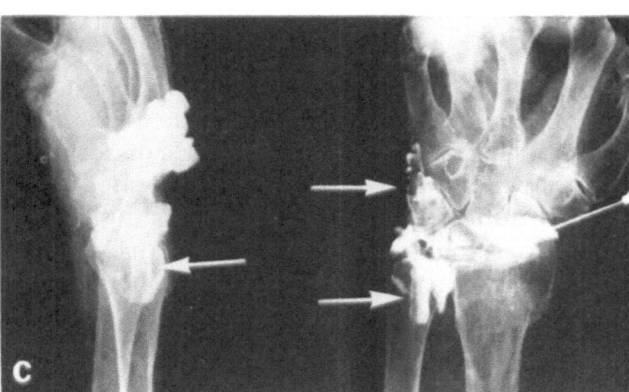

Fig. 4-1. **A.** The radiocarpal joint is demonstrated by arthrography. The pisicuneiform joint has not been filled. The arrow points to the prestyloid recess. **B.** The wrist joint communicates with the pisicuneiform joint in this case. The main synovial cavity lies over the ulnar styloid process. **C.** Arthrography of the radiocarpal joint. The pisicuneiform joint and the inferior radiocarpal joint have been filled at the same time. The sheath of extensor carpi ulnaris is filled also (arrows). (*From Weston and Kelsey: Br J Radiol 46:692, 1973.*)

sicuneiform joint, and the sheath of extensor carpi ulnaris, lies on the medial aspect of the wrist (Fig. 4-1A–C).

It is worth noting that in the normal wrist the skin contour on the flexor aspect of the wrist is concave (Fig. 4-3). The principal soft tissue landmark in the radiologic examination of the wrist region is the fatty plane which lies on the ventral aspect of pronator quadratus. This fat represents in part the extrasynovial fat of the sheaths of flexor sublimus and flexor profundus digitorum. The remainder of the fat forms the intermuscular fatty layer. Weinstein (35), in a small pamphlet, described the translucent line which may be seen in the lateral view of the wrist ventral to pronator quadratus. He

The Wrist and Hand

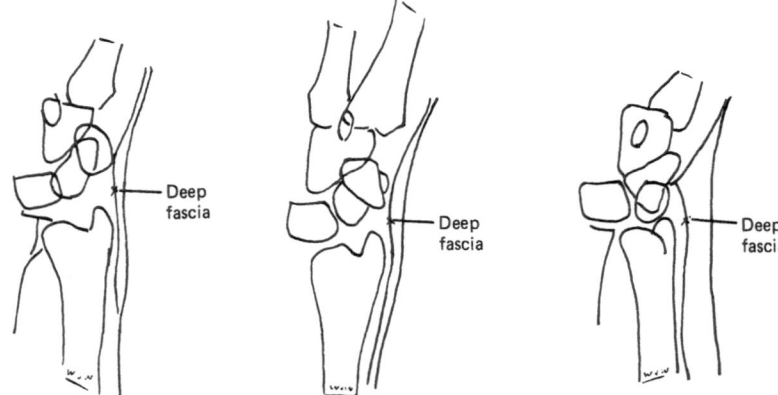

Fig. 4-2. Line diagram showing the normal variations of the relationship of the deep fascia to the ulnar styloid process. (*From Weston: Australas Radiol 12:384, 1968.*)

claimed this could be seen in 80 percent of normal wrists (Fig. 4-3). MacEwan (19) discussed the changes due to trauma in the fat plane overlying pronator quadratus. He dissected the forearm of a cadaver and noted that when he rotated off the tendons of flexor sublimus and flexor profundus digitorum a layer of fat was also rotated off pronator quadratus. Another fat plane just anterior to this was found to lie between the tendons of flexor profundus digitorum and the muscle mass of flexor sublimus digitorum.

When the normal wrist is studied arthrographically it is apparent that in only a small percentage of cases does the inferior radioulnar joint communicate with the wrist joint (Fig. 4-4), although Kaplan (12) considered there to be a com-

Fig. 4-3. The fat pad over pronator quadratus is well seen (arrows). It varies in thickness and may be double.

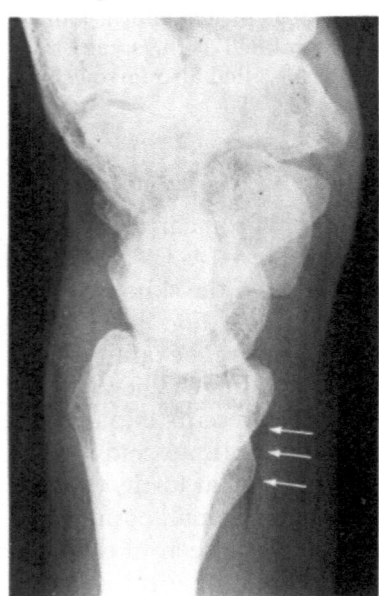

Fig. 4-4. Normal arthrogram showing a communication of the wrist joint with the inferior radioulnar joint. The latter joint cavity is convex centrally. **A** is anteroposterior view of arthrogram and **B** is lateral view.

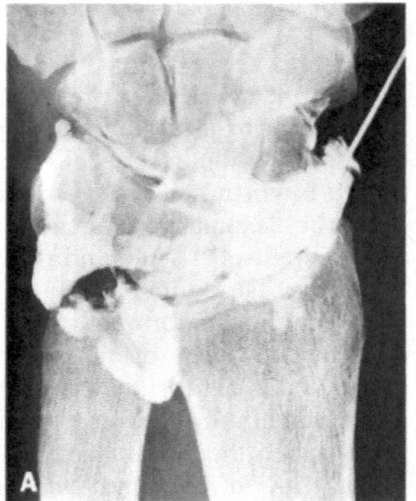
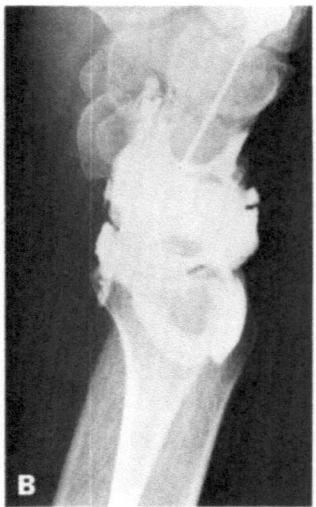

Soft Tissues of the Extremities

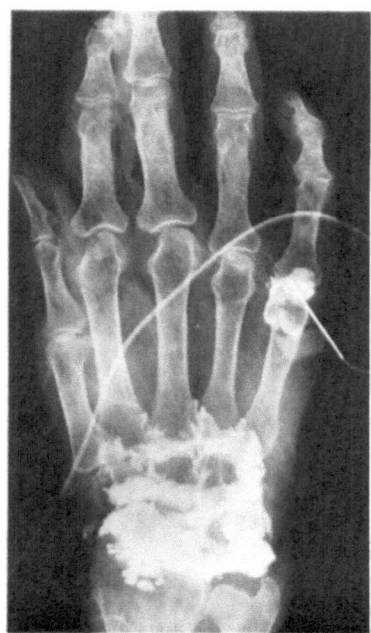

Fig. 4-5. The wrist joint may communicate with the intercarpal and carpometacarpal joints.

Fig. 4-6. Partial flexion of the wrist joint has produced a forward movement of the pisiform on the cuneiform. (*From Weston and Kelsey: Br J Radiol 46:692, 1973.*)

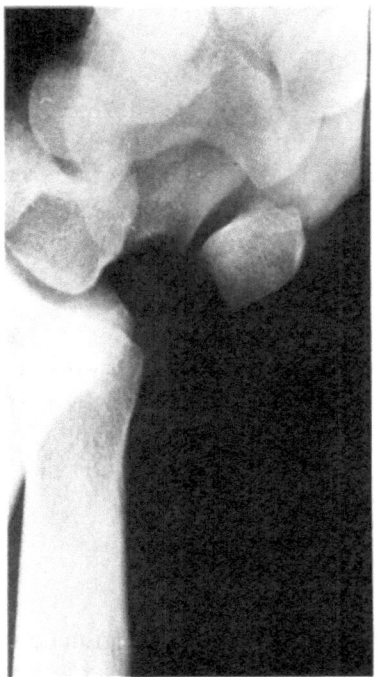

munication in 40 percent of cases. The wrist joint may communicate with the intercarpal and carpometacarpal joints (Fig. 4-5). Involvement of these joints by the rheumatoid process may contribute to the synovial mass arising from the carpus. It is also of interest that the wrist joint has been found to communicate with the pisicuneiform joint in 34 percent of cases. The "ball-catcher's" view of the wrist may be of value in assessing involvement of the latter.

THE PISICUNEIFORM JOINT

Anatomic texts (8,30) have usually described the pisicuneiform joint as a separate entity with a separate synovial cavity. The capsular ligaments surrounding the joint have been described as being attached to the edges of the opposed articular surfaces.

The tendon of flexor carpi ulnaris peripheral to the pisiform is continued on as the pisohamate and pisimetacarpal ligaments. A series of postmortem arthrograms of the wrist showed that the pisicuneiform joint was continuous with the radiocarpal joint in a number of cases. A large synovial cavity was noted both medial and distal to the articular surface of the pisiform. This is indirect evidence that this joint has either a redundant capsule or else a deficient capsule. It has been suggested by Wood Jones that the form of this joint cavity may be due to the pisiform being one of the lost digits, ie, postminimus.

When the wrist is flexed the pisiform first tilts on the cuneiform at its central articular margin (Fig. 4-6), and then moves in a ventral direction by about 2 to 3 mm when flexion with ulnar deviation is maximal (Fig. 4-7) (43). When this movement was first seen, subluxation or dislocation was considered as a possible cause, but when comparative views were taken of the normal wrist the movement was noted to be bilateral. This observation also supported the suggestion that the capsule of this joint is either larger than accepted by anatomists or is deficient.

Before subluxation or dislocation of the pisiform can be diagnosed the normal functional anatomy of this joint must be understood. When the normal wrist is fully extended the pisiform slides in a peripheral direction on the cuneiform and also rotates on its peripheral articular margin (Fig. 4-8).

In the supine oblique view, the so-called ball catcher's view, the tendon of flexor carpi ulnaris is shown to lie on the ventral aspect of the pisiform (5). This is similar to the respective positions of the tendon of quadriceps and the patella and is further reason why tilting can take place at the pisicuneiform joint. It also explains why a calcific tendinitis involving flexor carpi ulnaris may be seen involving the ven-

The Wrist and Hand

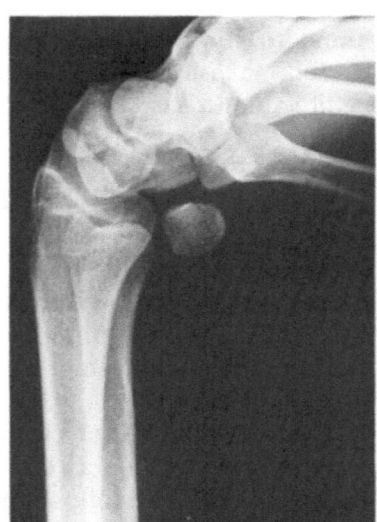

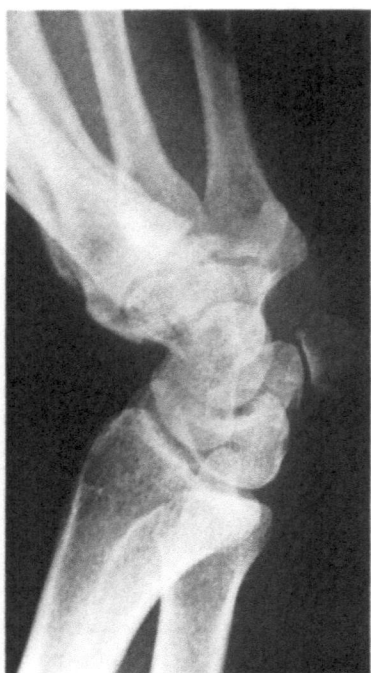

Fig. 4-7. Full flexion of the wrist joint. An apparent subluxation of the pisiform, which has become tilted. This movement is possible because of the lax synovial membrane and capsule. (*From Weston and Kelsey: Br J Radiol 46:692, 1973.*)

Fig. 4-8. Hyperextension of the wrist has produced tilting of the pisiform on the cuneiform at its peripheral articular margin. The joint space is widened centrally. (*From Weston and Kelsey: Br J Radiol 46:692, 1973.*)

tral aspect of the pisiform. It is the anatomy of flexor carpi ulnaris that determines the functional anatomy of the pisi-cuneiform joint and the relationship of the tendinitis calcarea to the pisiform (Fig. 4-9).

THE CARPOMETACARPAL JOINT OF THE THUMB

The carpometacarpal joint is saddle-shaped and it is not an easy joint to puncture percutaneously. The synovial cavity of this joint is also saddle-shaped (Fig. 4-10).

THE SYNOVIAL SHEATHS OF THE FLEXOR TENDONS OF THE WRIST

Contrast studies of the tendon sheaths of the wrist region contribute greatly to the appreciation of the soft tissue changes

Fig. 4-9. This line diagram shows the relationship of the tendon of flexor carpi ulnaris to the pisiform and cuneiform. The main bulk of the pisiform lies dorsal to the tendon of flexor carpi ulnaris. A similar situation is seen at the patella.

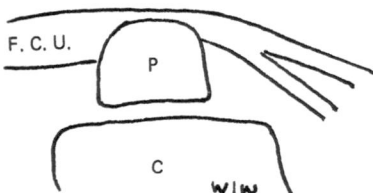

Soft Tissues of the Extremities

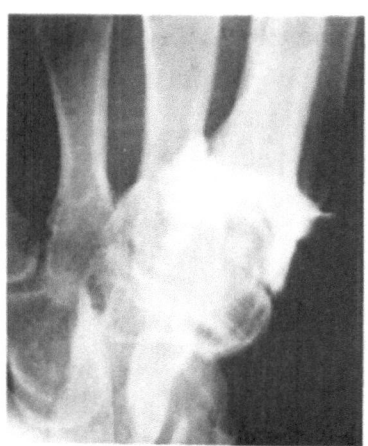

Fig. 4-10. A postmortem arthrogram of the carpometacarpal joint of the thumb. The joint cavity is saddle-shaped.

in disease. Weston (42) described the contrast-filled ulnar bursa, which forms a common sheath for the tendons of flexor sublimus digitorum and flexor profundus digitorum. The sheath extends 2.5 cm above the anterior carpal ligament (1,10) and downward to the midpalm (Fig. 4-11A and B).

Scheldrup (32) demonstrated the variable pattern of termination of the ulnar bursa in 367 postmortem dissections. A summary of the findings is shown in Figure 4-12. Normally the tendons of flexor sublimus digitorum and flexor profundus digitorum converge on the carpal tunnel, rather like a half-opened fan.

The radial bursa about flexor pollicis longus can also be outlined by injection of the sheath of this bursa at the level of the proximal phalanx of the thumb. The tip of a 21-gauge butterfly needle is placed in contact with the midshaft of the proximal phalanx of the thumb and the contrast media injected (Fig. 4-13A and B). Similarly, the sheath of flexor carpi radialis can be injected percutaneously above the anterior carpal ligament and lateral to the tendon of palmaris longus.

SOFT TISSUE CHANGES OF THE WRIST REGION

Acute Nonspecific Tenosynovitis

Acute nonspecific tenosynovitis may produce a striking radiographic pattern in the soft tissues. Edema is noted on the dorsolateral aspect of the lower third of the forearm. This edema disrupts the fascia–fat interface and causes the thickened septae that are seen joining the deep fascia to the cutis line. These septae are interlinked by further septae that run in the long axis of the forearm.

Stenosing Tenovaginitis or de Quervain's Disease

In 1895 de Quervain (23) described a condition affecting the tendons of abductor pollicis longus and extensor pollicis brevis at the radial styloid process. A good description of the condition is to be found in *Gray's Anatomy* (9) under the name of "washer woman's sprain."

Continued friction between the tendon, tendon sheath, and the radial styloid process leads to edema of the sheath and an increase in fluid may be present within it. This is a reversible stage; but it may be followed by fibrosis in the tendon sheath which may be thickened to 3 or 4 mm. This condition can be diagnosed radiologically and it is important for a radiologist to recognize the changes when the more obvious clinical signs have been overlooked.

Burman (6) made an extensive review of the literature.

The Wrist and Hand

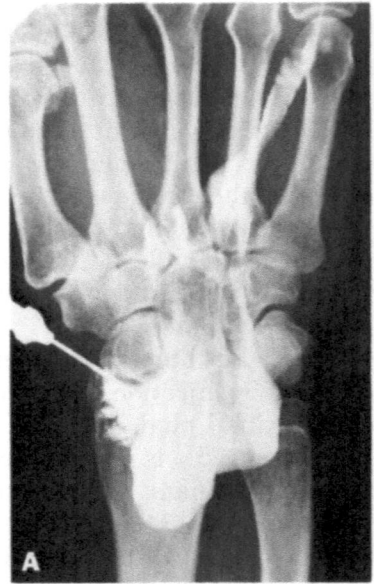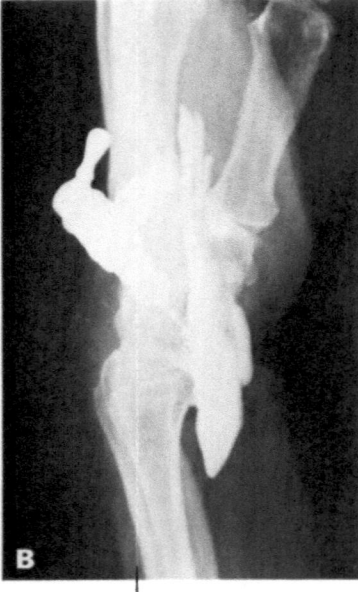

Fig. 4-11. Anteroposterior **(A)** and lateral **(B)** radiographs of the ulnar bursa injected with 5 ml of barium sulfate at postmortem examination. The bursa is continuous with the digital sheath about the tendon of flexor sublimis digitorum and flexor profundus digitorum to the little finger. (*From Weston: Australas Radiol 17:216, 1973.*)

Lewis (17) stated that de Quervain's disease is readily recognized radiologically in well-developed cases by a rather localized soft tissue swelling that obscures the shadows of the adjacent tendons. Weston (36) described 47 cases of this condition. The soft tissue signs are best studied under three headings (Fig. 4-14A and B). There were no changes in the underlying bone.

Deformity of the Cutis Line Because of the swelling of the tendon sheath which may or may not contain fluid, the cutis line is deformed by a convex bulge laterally.

Thickening of the Tendon Sheath Complex The tendon, tendon sheath, and synovial fluid cannot be separated and thus the soft tissue shadow of the tendon sheath complex is thicker than usual. The tendon sheath has an outer fatty extrasynovial layer which defines its margin clearly. Its lateral margin is also defined by the fascia–subcutaneous fat interface. When abductor pollicis longus and extensor pollicis brevis have separate sheaths, one may see two thickened tendon sheath complexes separated by a fine line of fat (Fig. 4-14A and B). This thickened mass varied from 2.5 to 5 cm in length over the radial styloid process and as it skirts the anatomist's snuff-box.

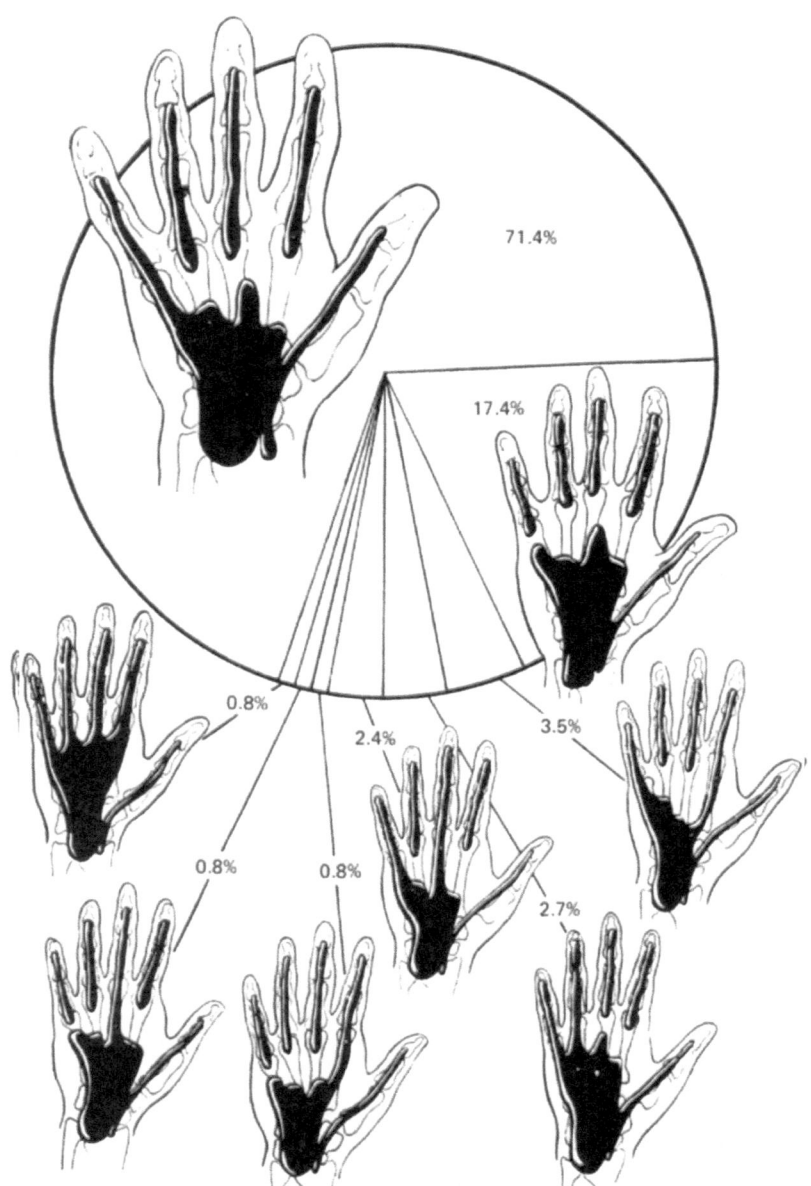

Fig. 4-12. Schematic diagram showing arrangements of the digital sheaths with respect to the palmar ganglion and the sheath of flexor longus pollicus. *(After Scheldrup: Mod Med 20:92, 1952.)*

Edema In the more acute cases edema can be noted on the outer side of the wrist with thickening of the cutis line in association with the two signs noted above.

Ganglion Formation

A ganglion is a circumscribed lesion which is usually oval or circular (Fig. 4-15). It can be differentiated from the sausage-shaped lesion of de Quervain's disease. If an at-

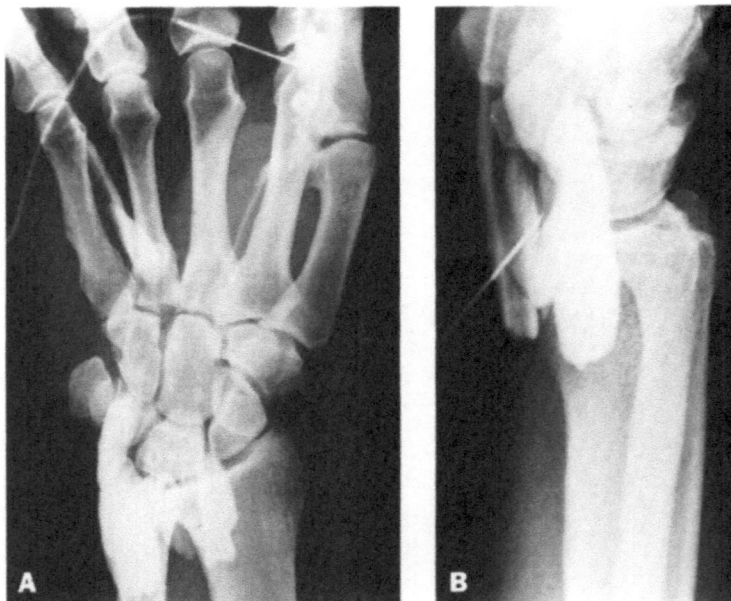

Fig. 4-13. Anteroposterior (**A**) and lateral (**B**) projections. The radial and ulnar bursae have been filled separately with barium sulfate at postmortem examination. The radial bursa lies ventral to the ulnar bursa.

Fig. 4-14. A. No bony lesion is detected. There is considerable thickening of the tendon sheath complex at the level of the radial styloid process (arrow). A thin line of fat in the mass indicates that two separate sheaths are involved. The cutis line is deformed over the mass. **B.** Line diagram demonstrating the thickened tendon sheath complex over the radial styloid process with deformed cutis line. The thin line of fat in this tendon complex indicates that two separate sheaths are involved: de Quervain's disease. (*From Weston: Br J Radiol 40:446, 1967.*)

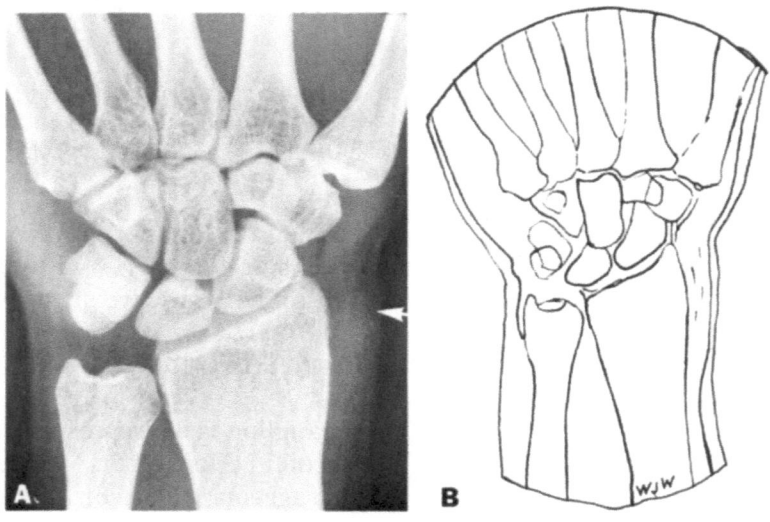

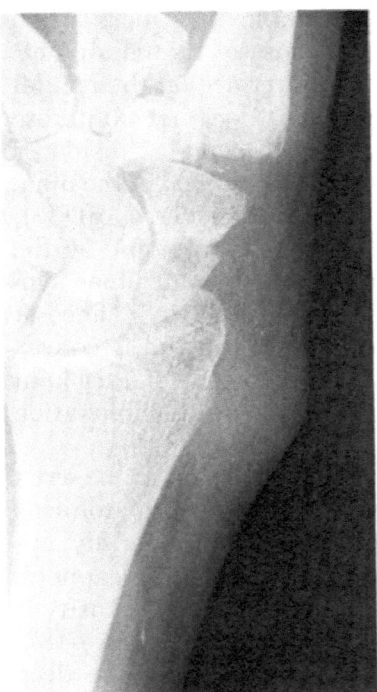

Fig. 4-15. A moderately large ganglion lies over the radial styloid process. The cutis line is deformed over the ganglion.

Fig. 4-16. A synovial mass lesion is present at the level of the ulnar styloid process due to rheumatoid involvement of the wrist joint (arrow). The mass lesion displaces the deep fascia away from the styloid process and causes the increased density.

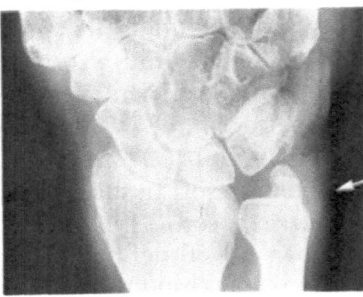

tempt is made to aspirate such a lesion the gelatinous contents are difficult to withdraw.

Other Lesions

Less commonly, an osteomyelitis of the radial styloid process causes edema in this area but no change in the tendon sheath complex. Furthermore, the underlying bone changes will usually be apparent. Tendon sheath tumors are extremely rare, but must be considered.

RHEUMATOID DISEASE OF THE WRIST

Lockie (18) stated that "The hand in rheumatoid arthritis characteristically shows involvement of the proximal interphalangeal joints and the metacarpophalangeal joints, as well as swelling of the ulnar side of the wrist. Also there may be fluid present in any of these involved joints and in the tendon sheaths of the back of the hand." Lewis (17,28) stated that "In the diagnosis of early rheumatoid arthritis study of the hands is particularly rewarding." Long before cartilage or bone destruction occurs there are three areas of soft tissue swelling which may announce the presence of the disease.

1. Fusiform soft tissue swelling about one or several proximal interphalangeal joints
2. Capsular distention of one or more metacarpophalangeal joints
3. Localized soft tissue swelling on the ulnar side of the wrist, about or just distal to the lower extremity of the ulna

If all three are present, the diagnosis of rheumatoid arthritis is nearly certain. If two are found, the disease is to be suspected; if one is seen in the absence of trauma the possibility of the disease should be considered.

Soila (33) discussed the soft tissue changes in the hand and wrist, but made no specific comment on the region of the ulnar styloid process. He made an extensive review of the literature, including the soft tissue changes. Martel et al (21) have described the erosive changes at the wrist and Martel (20) noted that subtle soft tissue thickening can often be seen at the wrist, particularly adjacent to the ulnar styloid process. Berens et al (3) stated that "The distal ulna may act as a beacon for the recognition of rheumatoid arthritis, early in the disease. The earliest changes to be found are soft tissue swelling medial to the head of ulna, which has a homogeneous water density obliterating the fascial–fat plane."

The changes around the ulnar styloid process are quite predictable and in our experience do not obliterate the fascia–fat

The Wrist and Hand

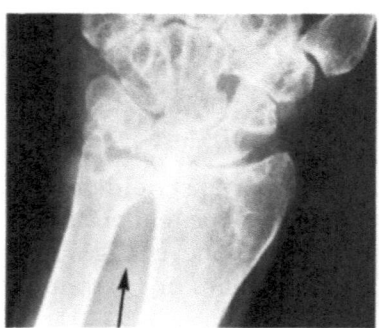

Fig. 4-17. Rheumatoid arthritis involving the wrist joint and inferior radioulnar joint. Two mass lesions are produced. That of the inferior radioulnar joint lies on the interosseous membrane proximal to the joint (arrow).

Fig. 4-18. With involvement of the wrist joint by rheumatoid arthritis one can see a synovial mass lying between the radial styloid process and the scaphoid bone (arrow). This mass is dense and extends into the anatomist's snuff-box.

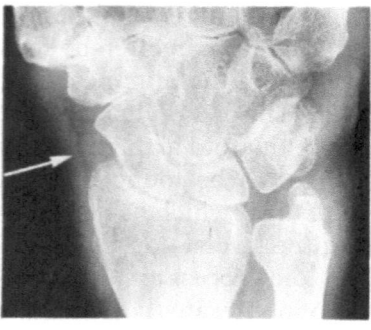

planes. The rheumatoid synovial complex is a mass lesion that is visible in the soft tissues because of its mass alone. Secondly, it displaces the fascia–fat interface on the medial aspect of the ulnar styloid process, but does not obliterate this interface. In this area the synovial complex displaces the deep fascia medially away from the lower end of the ulna, the ulnar styloid process, and the cuneiform (Fig. 4-16) (37).

The involvement of the inferior radioulnar joint by the rheumatoid process is the precursor of the caput ulnae syndrome (2). The synovial mass lesion is also easily defined at the lower end of the interosseous membrane and is convex centrally (Fig. 4-17). Soft tissue involvement of this joint gives the initial warning of the possible future subluxation and dislocation of this joint.

In a number of cases, the synovial mass lesion at the wrist can also be seen on close inspection of the anatomist's snuff-box. A mass lesion, which is convex peripherally, appears between the lower end of the radius and the scaphoid. It encroaches on the anatomist's snuff-box and its density is continuous with that of the radius and scaphoid (Fig. 4-18).

In acute cases one sees both displacement of the deep fascia together with disruption of the fascia–fat interface due to edema. This, too, is often best seen at the level of the ulnar styloid process (Fig. 4-19).

The fat line seen on the lateral view of the wrist, over pronator quadratus, may provide a useful early radiologic sign of wrist involvement in rheumatoid arthritis, although, as noted by Weinstein (35), "this has received almost no mention in the literature. The pronator quadratus fat line becomes indistinct in some cases and in others it has merely been displaced or bowed by the underlying inflammatory swelling. Occasionally it has been possible to demonstrate return of the fat line once the active phase has subsided, and the disease has become quiescent."

Soft tissue swelling at the wrist may also be due to involvement of one or more of the tendon sheaths in the region. Swelling of the sheaths of flexor carpi ulnaris and flexor carpi radialis may be seen on the medial and lateral aspects of the wrist joint, respectively, while on the dorsum of the hand effusion into the common extensor sheath may be visible in a lateral view. On the ventral aspect a mass lesion is produced when the ulnar bursa itself is involved in rheumatoid arthritis. This results from edema fluid, synovial fluid, synovial hypertrophy, and perhaps melon-seed bodies. This ventral mass has been demonstrated at operation and is well illustrated in a photograph from the book by Flatt (7) (Fig. 4-20). It can be studied in the plain film when the soft tissues in the lateral view of the wrist are not overexposed (41,42). The mass lesion is sausage-shaped and has a well-defined proximal pole (Fig. 4-21A and B). Its shape corresponds to that

Soft Tissues of the Extremities

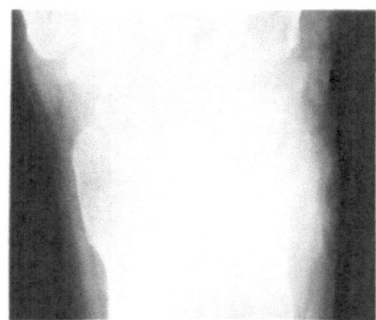

Fig. 4-19. In acute cases of rheumatoid arthritis one may see a synovial mass lesion over the ulnar styloid process. This causes fascial displacement. The edema causes disruption of the fascia–fat interface.

Fig. 4-20. The cystic masses in rheumatoid arthritis which may be found along the tendons of flexor sublimis digitorum and flexor profundus digitorum at operation are shown. (*After Flatt: The Care of the Rheumatoid Hand, 1968. Courtesy of Mosby.*)

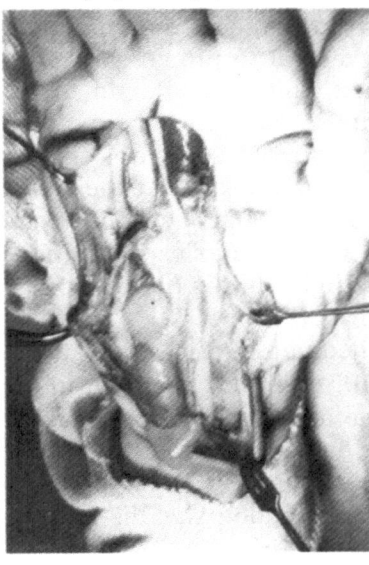

seen in postmortem injections of the normal sheath, and to that of the contrast-filled ulnar bursa involved by the rheumatoid process (Fig. 4-22A and B).

The synovial mass lesion about the tendon increases the soft tissue density which can be seen even when fast film and screens have been used. Normally, in the lateral view, the ventral aspect of the lower end of the forearm is concave, but when the ulnar bursa is enlarged it becomes convex and the

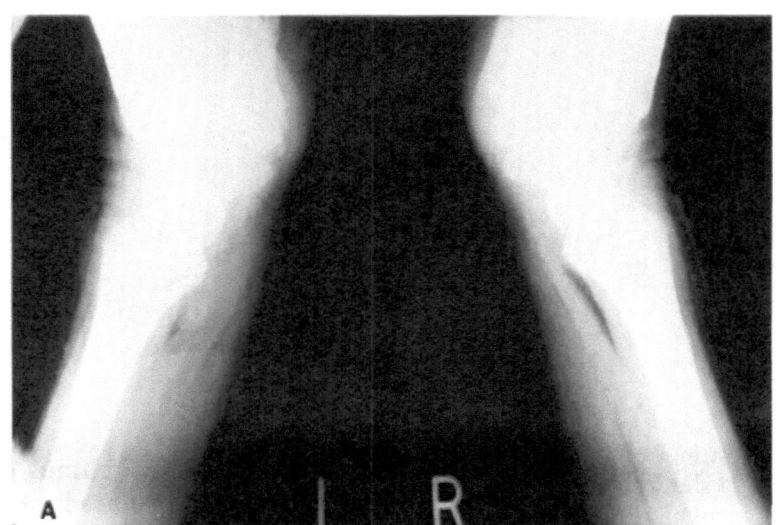

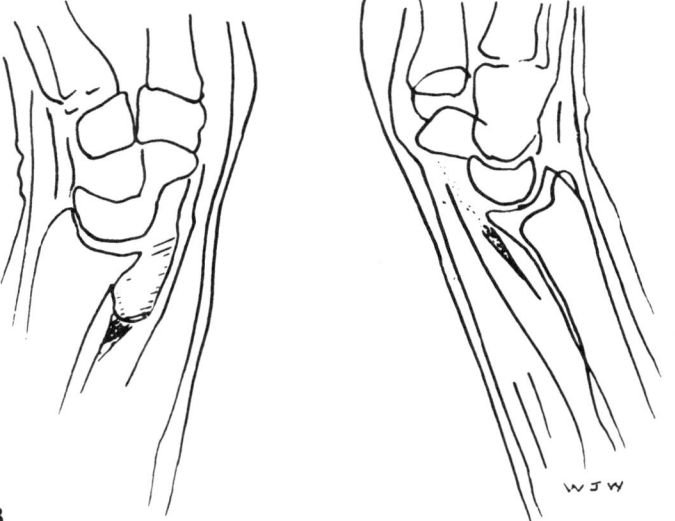

Fig. 4-21. **A.** Lateral soft tissue views of the affected wrist and the normal wrist. The displaced extrasynovial fat in the affected ulnar bursa is reduced in length, increased in thickness, and has a concave base directed to the wrist. **B.** Line diagram of **A**. (*From Weston: J Can Assoc Radiol 24:282, 1973.*)

The Wrist and Hand

Fig. 4-22. The opaque medium in the ulnar bursa has passed through the hourglass constriction caused by the carpal ligament into a dilated sheath within the palm. Anteroposterior (**A**) and lateral (**B**) views.

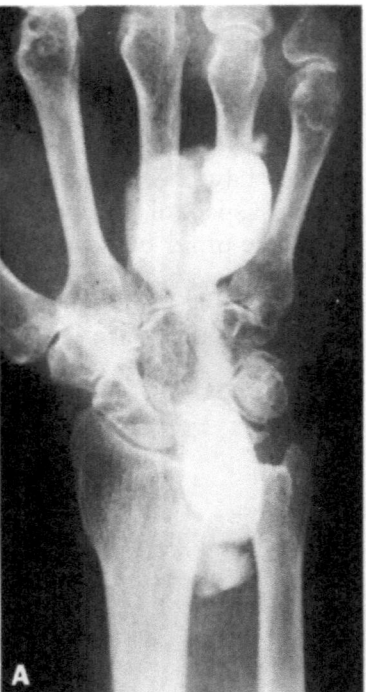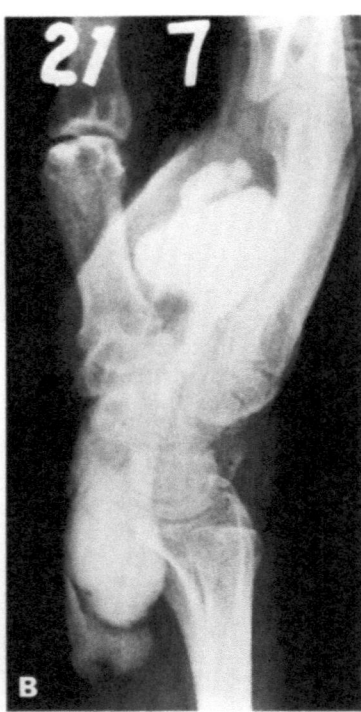

Fig. 4-23. Arthrography of the wrist in rheumatoid disease may show deep erosions of articular surfaces and nodular hypertrophic changes of the synovium. Communication with the inferior radioulnar joint and tendon sheath of extensor carpi ulnaris may also be demonstrated. (*From Palmer: Ann Intern Med 70:61, 1969.*)

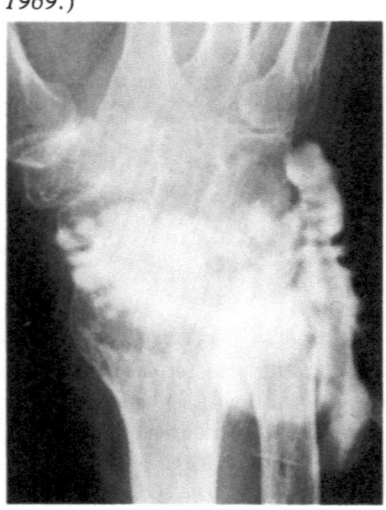

tendons of flexor sublimus digitorum and flexor profundus digitorum are displaced forward. This increases the thickness of the soft tissue ventral to the radius and a gentle hump appears that interrupts the normal smooth skin contour. This change is easier to appreciate if one has the opposite limb for comparison, as the thickness of the normal soft tissues varies from person to person. When both sides are involved, one may be able to refer back to earlier serial films.

When the ulnar bursa is involved in the rheumatoid process the extrasynovial fatty pad ventral to pronator quadratus becomes shortened, thickened, and triangular in shape. The apex of the triangle points toward the elbow, with the concave base toward the wrist. This is very similar in form to the intrasynovial fatty changes seen at the elbow which were first described by Norrell (22). The thin strip of fat normally seen between the tendons of flexor sublimus digitorum and flexor profundus digitorum is obliterated by the synovial mass lesion.

Arthrography of the wrist in rheumatoid disease is likely to reveal greater damage to the joint than that apparent in the plain film. Deep erosions of the articular surfaces may be outlined and the typical nodular hypertrophic changes of the synovium are seen in silhouette (Fig. 4-23) (27). Communications with various involved tendon sheaths may be demonstrated.

Soft Tissues of the Extremities

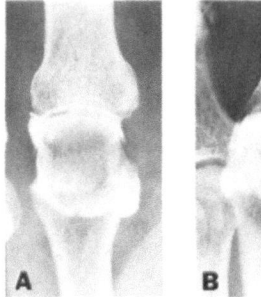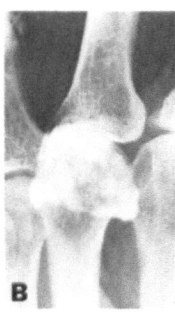
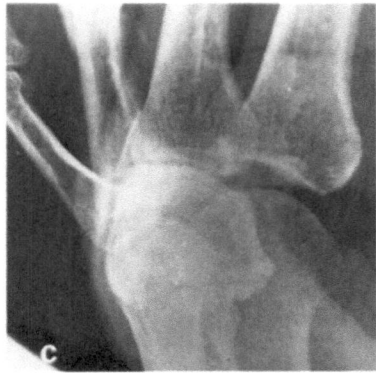

Fig. 4-24. Postmortem arthrogram of a normal metacarpophalangeal joint. Posteroanterior (**A**), oblique (**B**), and lateral (**C**) projections. The waist seen in the posteroanterior view is produced by the collateral ligaments. (*From Weston: Australas Radiol 13:211, 1969.*)

RADIOLOGIC ANATOMY OF THE HAND

The best anatomic description of the synovial cavities of the metacarpophalangeal and interphalangeal joints was found to be that of Testut and Jacob (34). The synovial membrane lining each of these joints was found to be reflected well back on the palmar aspects of the heads and necks of the metacarpals and phalanges, respectively.

The synovial membrane of the metacarpophalangeal joint is attached to the articular margin of the head of the metacarpal. Most of the synovial membrane lies on the ventral aspect of the head and neck of the metacarpal. The articular surfaces of the metacarpal heads are broader in front than behind. The capsule is loosely attached to the ventral aspect of the metacarpal. It is firmly attached to the base of the proximal phalanx close to the articular surface.

Postmortem arthrography (39) can be performed with the metacarpophalangeal or interphalangeal joint flexed to a right angle. The joint space is then easily palpated on the dorsal aspect of the joint on either side of the extensor tendon. Once the space is located, a 26-gauge needle is inserted through the extensor expansion, which fixes the needle. As the opaque medium enters the joint, the synovial cavity is distended. This can be palpated by the left index finger of the operator, which is placed on the palmar aspect of the joint. The distended cavity is tense and cystic and it displaces the index finger away from the metacarpal head. An alternative technique, with the finger held in extension, consists of inserting the needle from the lateral aspect between the extensor apparatus dorsally and the articular surfaces ventrally.

The opaque medium within the metacarpophalangeal joint is seen as a thin layer over the head of the metacarpal and between the metacarpal head and phalanx. On the lateral aspects of the joint the small recess has a waist due to the collateral ligaments. A large recess is noted on the palmar aspect of the metacarpal head and neck. This extends proximally about 1 cm from the joint space (Fig. 4-24A–C). The metacarpophalangeal joint of the thumb is shown in Figure 4-25A and B.

The anatomy of the joint space explains why the distended synovial cavity of the joint is visualized proximal to the joint line. As the largest component is on the palmar aspect of the joint, it can be appreciated that this aspect is not seen to advantage in the standard posteroanterior views taken in routine investigation of cases of possible rheumatoid arthritis.

Within the proximal interphalangeal joints of the fingers the opaque medium is seen as a thin layer between the head of the proximal phalanx, with its two condyles, and the dou-

The Wrist and Hand

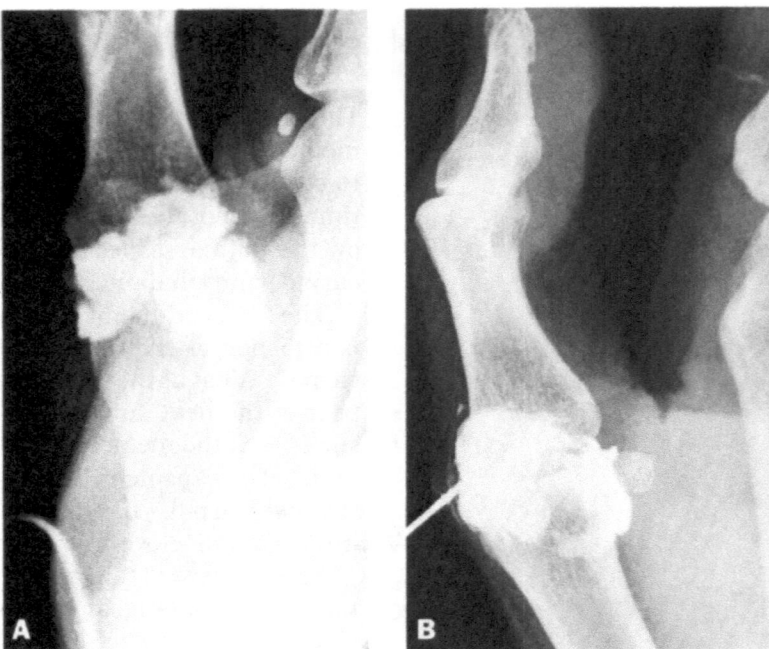

Fig. 4-25. Postmortem arthrogram of the metacarpophalangeal joint of the thumb. Posteroanterior (**A**) and oblique (**B**) projections. (*From Weston: Australas Radiol 13:211, 1969.*)

Fig. 4-26. Posteroanterior (**A**) and lateral (**B**) views of an arthrogram of the proximal interphalangeal joint of a finger. Note double facets on the base of the intermediate phalanx. (*From Weston: Australas Radiol 13:211, 1969.*)

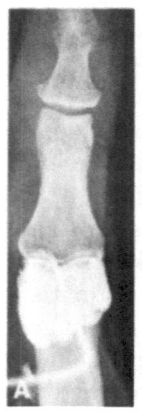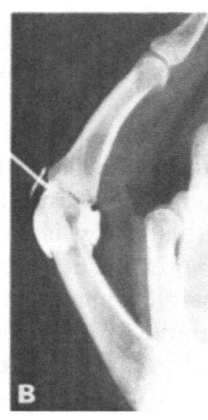

ble facet seen on the base of the intermediate phalanx (Fig. 4-26A and B). The shape of the synovial cavity is similar to that seen in the metacarpophalangeal joints. The opaque medium shows a waist on the lateral and medial aspects of the joint, due to the collateral ligaments. The synovial cavity extends up the palmar aspect of the neck of the proximal phalanx for about 7 mm.

An arthrogram of the distal interphalangeal joint is shown in Figure 4-27A and B. It will be noted that in the distal interphalangeal joint the dorsal component of the joint recess is almost as large as the ventral one, and the synovial cavity is almost H-shaped.

In the normal finger in the posteroanterior view one can see the margins of the fibrous portions of the fibroosseous tunnels that constitute the digital tendon sheaths. These run parallel to the neck and shaft of the proximal and intermediate phalanges and extend about 1 mm lateral to the cortex of the phalanx. At the level of the joint one finds the capsule of the joint enclosed by the fibrous tunnel, and thus one sees a normal spindle-shaped contour of the fibroosseous canal at the level of the proximal and distal interphalangeal joints.

Tenosynography may be undertaken by introducing contrast medium into the digital sheath through a needle inserted both centrally and centrifugally through the palmar aspect of the base of the finger. The surface marking is the

Soft Tissues of the Extremities

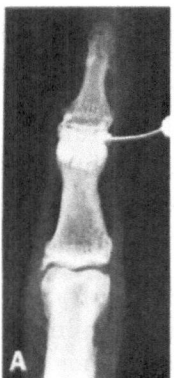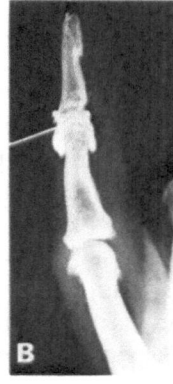

Fig. 4-27. Arthrogram of the distal interphalangeal joint in posteroanterior **(A)** and lateral **(B)** projections. *(From Weston: Australas Radiol 13:211, 1969.)*

Fig. 4-28. A. The common sheath of flexor sublimus digitorum and flexor profundus digitorum is demonstrated. **B.** The accumulation of the contrast material about the reflection of the digital sheaths at the level of the neck of the metacarpal is shown (arrow). *(From Weston: Australas Radiol 13:211, 1969.)*

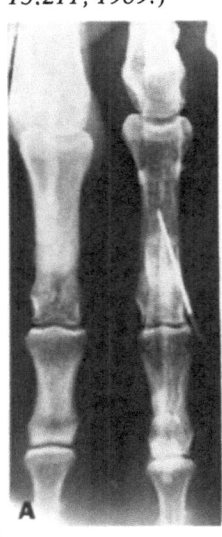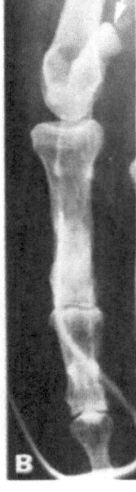

distal crease at the base of the finger, where it joins the hand. The orifice of the 21 scalp vein needle is inserted parallel to the long axis of the phalanx until the tip is just touching bone in the region of the base of the proximal phalanx.

The palmar prolongation of the synovial membrane of the proximal interphalangeal joint is missed by this technique, ie, central insertion. The needle must be in the midline of the finger.

When the cavity of the sheath is entered, there is no delay of the entry of the contrast medium into the sheath and its passage peripherally can be seen and palpated. The sheaths can be adequately outlined by 0.5 to 0.6 ml of 60 percent hypaque (29,38). A knowledge of the normal anatomy and the normal pattern seen with positive contrast agents is essential to the medical or surgical management of tenosynovitis and tendon nodules.

The anatomic pattern of the communication of the digital sheaths with the radial and ulnar bursae has been described by Resnick (25) and Scheldrup (32). The tendons of flexor sublimus digitorum and flexor profundus digitorum have a common sheath in the fibroosseous tunnel in the fingers (Fig. 4-28A). The synovial sheath in the average case ceases in the palm just proximal to the metacarpal head. The reflection of the tendon sheath is accentuated by a small accumulation of contrast medium at this point (Fig. 4-28B). The contrast surrounds and outlines the tendons which appear as cylindrical, space-occupying masses in both diameters (Fig. 4-29). The synovial sheaths show small folds in the anteroposterior view, and these are best seen near the joints (Fig. 4-30A and B). The insertion of flexor sublimus digitorum at the base of the intermediate phalanx is clearly shown as the tendon assumes a crescentic shape where it traverses the convex capsule of the proximal interphalangeal joint (26). The tendon of insertion of flexor profundus digitorum into the base of the terminal phalanx shows the same pattern and is well outlined by contrast. The digital sheath for the little finger communicates with the ulnar bursa in 71.4 percent of cases according to Scheldrup (32). The digital sheath in the thumb communicates with the sheath about the tendon of flexor pollicis longus in 100 percent of cases, ie, the radial bursa.

Soft Tissue Changes

Widening of the joint space can be seen with intracapsular fractures of the metacarpophalangeal, metatarsophalangeal, and interphalangeal joints of the hand and foot in children. This does not happen in all cases with intracapsular fractures, but can be a useful indirect sign of that condition (Fig. 4-31A and B) (40).

A working hypothesis is that this widening is due to he-

The Wrist and Hand

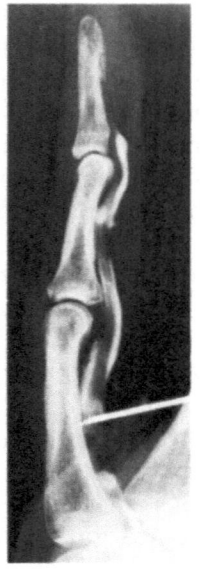

Fig. 4-29. The tendons of flexor sublimus digitorum and flexor profundus digitorum form a cylindrical filling defect in the tendon sheath. The tendons at their insertions assume a crescentic shape where they traverse the convex capsules of the proximal and distal interphalangeal joints. (*From Weston: Australas Radiol 13:211, 1969.*)

marthrosis. For this to actually be the case, two possibilities must be considered.

1. An intact joint capsule with an intracapsular fracture
2. An intact joint capsule with an intracapsular fracture reaching the periosteum: the periosteum may strip off the bone but remains intact

Kittleson and Whitehouse (13) and Salter (31) both mention that the periosteal tube is thick and resistant in children, and this could explain the radiographic findings when the fracture line separates off a bony fragment but leaves the joint space distended. The thick periosteal tube remains intact even though a fragment of bone has been separated off the parent bone. This means that the intact joint cavity becomes continuous with the space formed by the fracture line bounded by the periosteal tube. After 2 to 3 weeks the joint width returns toward normal and early callus formation will be seen at the fracture site.

Mucoid cysts have been found adjacent to both the proximal interphalangeal and distal interphalangeal joints, although two studies (4,14) described these lesions in relation to the distal interphalangeal joints only (Fig. 4-32).

Direct trauma to a finger may produce a hematoma in the flexor sheath. When the digital sheath is separate from the ulnar bursa, a tense collection of fluid can form. The finger is enlarged and the fibroosseous tunnel is distended, acting as a space-occupying lesion. Tuberculosis of the tendon sheaths

Fig. 4-30. Small folds are shown in the tendon sheath near the level of the interphalangeal joints. Contrast injected into flexor sheaths at P.M. **A** is anteroposterior view. **B** is oblique view of these sheaths. (*From Weston: Australas Radiol 13:360, 1969.*)

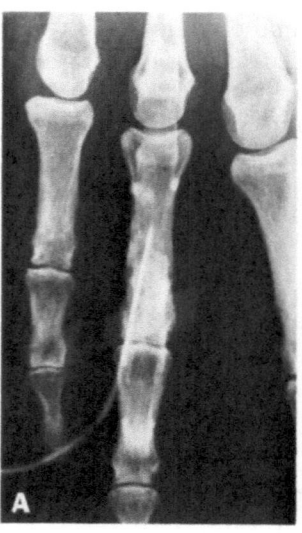
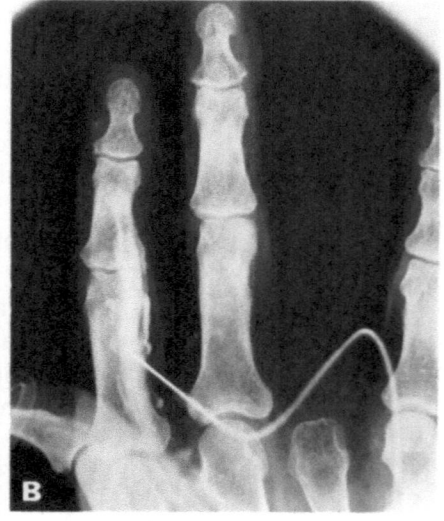

Soft Tissues of the Extremities

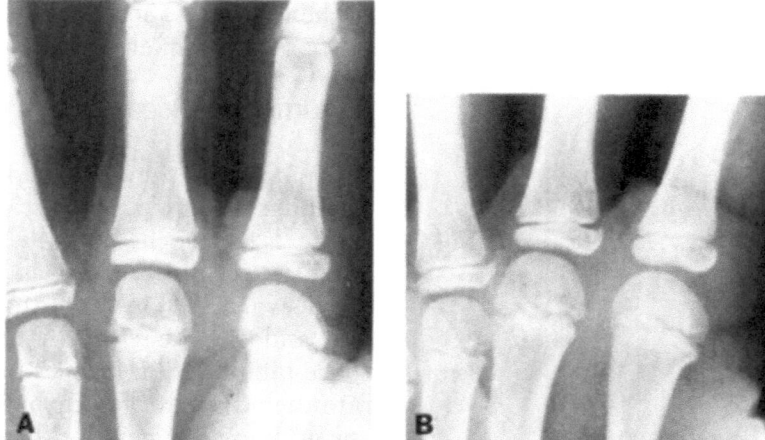

Fig. 4-31. Anteroposterior **(A)** and oblique **(B)** views of the right hand with an intracapsular fracture of the head of the second right metacarpal associated with joint space widening. (*From Weston: Australas Radiol 15:367, 1971.*)

Fig. 4-32. A mucoid cyst may cause a localized swelling adjacent to an interphalangeal joint.

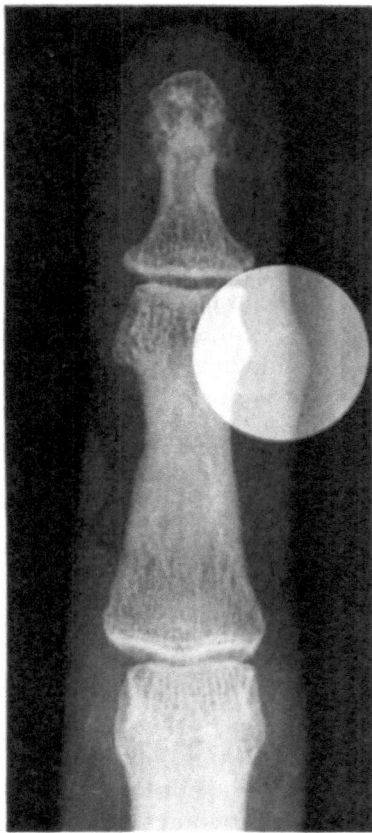

Fig. 4-33. A synovial mass lesion due to rheumatoid arthritis is seen about the metacarpophalangeal joint (arrows). The increased density is a striking feature and a "shoulder" is present at the level of the base of the proximal phalanx.

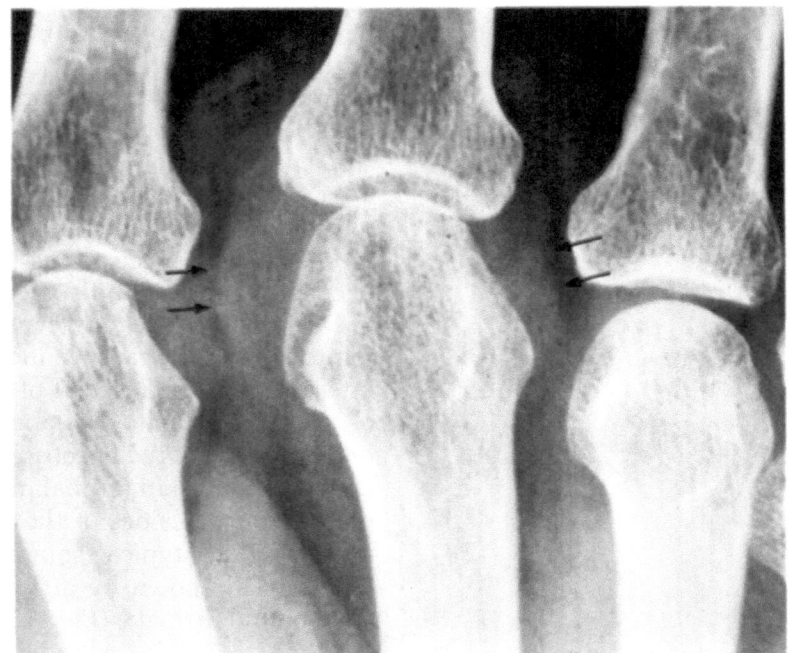

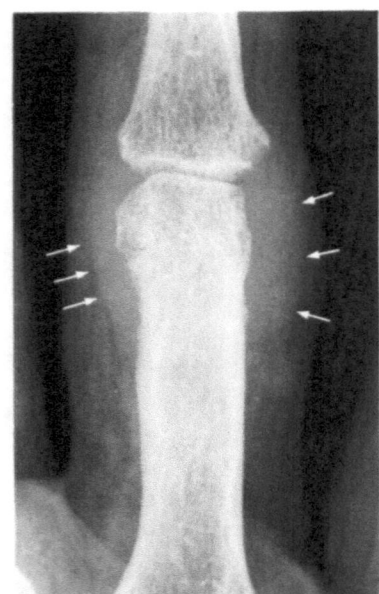

Fig. 4-34. The synovial mass is seen about a proximal interphalangeal joint. The mass lesions are denser than the normal tissues. The mass is wider than the normal pattern of soft tissues about a proximal interphalangeal joint and produces a spindle-shaped swelling (arrows).

of the fingers is another cause of a mass lesion distending the fibroosseous tunnel, and must enter the differential diagnosis.

Rheumatoid Disease

The pattern of the distended interphalangeal or metacarpophalangeal joint is similar, whether it is seen with trauma, septic arthritis, hemophilia, rheumatoid disease, or allied conditions.

The waist seen in the normal metacarpophalangeal joint is lost and the distended joint becomes rounded off. The space-taking lesion formed by the distended joint may separate the adjacent metacarpal heads. This is most conspicuous with involvement by rheumatoid arthritis. The mass lesion so produced in rheumatoid disease runs from the base of the proximal phalanx down to the neck of the metacarpal. The smooth capsule is replaced by a distinct hump or shoulder starting from the base of the proximal phalanx (Fig. 4-33). The mass lesion shows an increased density. Normally, one can usually see a strip of fat parallel with the metacarpal head lying between the capsules of the metacarpophalangeal joints. As the metacarpophalangeal joint enlarges the fat strip becomes narrowed and finally lost.

The main portion of the distended synovial cavity of the metacarpophalangeal joint is seen proximal to the joint line in the posteroanterior view of the hand. The larger component on the palmar aspect of the joint is not, however, seen to advantage in this view. In lateral views the distended joint cavity is also well seen on the dorsal aspect of these joints. Similar findings are noted in views obtained with the fingers flexed using a tangential beam and the closed fist in contact with the film.

In the case of the second metacarpophalangeal joint the mass lesion can be seen displacing the deep fascia of the first web space. Instead of the soft tissues being concave in this area, they become convex. The first metacarpophalangeal joint is obtained as a true lateral and the normal waist seen on the dorsal aspect of this joint becomes lost. The capsule becomes convex and displaces the deep fascia dorsally.

Disease processes involving the proximal interphalangeal joints distend the capsule and become visible on the lateral or lateral and medial aspects of the joint. A shoulder at the base of the intermediate phalanx is formed (Fig. 4-34). The fibrous portion of the fibroosseous tunnel is displaced from the neck of the proximal phalanx. Finally the cutis line is displaced on both sides of the proximal interphalangeal joint, producing the typical spindle-shaped deformity. This pattern is well shown by arthrography of a joint involved by rheumatoid arthritis (Fig. 4.35A and B). The anatomy of the joint space explains why the distended synovial cavity of the

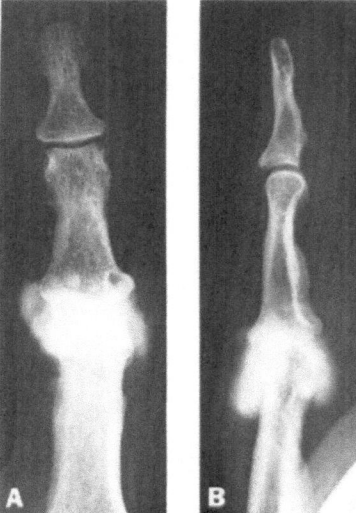

Fig. 4-35. Arthrograms of a proximal interphalangeal joint involved by rheumatoid arthritis. The enlarged joint cavity is a typical finding.
A. Posterior-antero view.
B. Lateral view.

proximal interphalangeal joint is seen in the main, proximal to the joint line in the posteroanterior view of the hand. The largest component is again on the palmar aspect of the joint, and is not seen to advantage in the standard posteroanterior views.

Rheumatoid arthritis may result in a fluid effusion into the flexor sheaths, thickening and irregularity of the synovium, and localized hypertrophy with the formation of a nodule and mechanical interference with movement. There may be loss of parallelism of the fibrous tunnel to the shafts of the proximal and intermediate phalanges, for these mass lesions can be eccentric to the shaft of the phalanx. In the lateral projection there is an increase in the thickness of the fibroosseous tunnel, which displaces the skin and subcutaneous fat in a palmar direction (Fig. 4-36A and B).

If the involved digital sheaths are instilled with urografin, the size of the tunnel is seen to be enlarged in both anteroposterior and lateral diameters. The coarse, nodular, and thick hypertrophic synovial membrane is outlined. It is of interest that the digital lymphatics may fill (Fig. 4-37) (5). This sign appears to be typical of rheumatoid disease. The contrast medium may not, however, outline the whole sheath owing to segmental blockages. Sometimes the proximal ends of the digital sheaths become sacculated with extensions that pass through the palmar fascia into the subcutaneous tissues (Fig. 4-38A and B).

Fig. 4-36. Anteroposterior **(A)** and lateral **(B)** views of the radiographs of a flexor nodule (arrows) in the finger. **C.** Line diagrams of **A** and **B**. The fibrous portion of the fibroosseous tunnel is deformed by the nodule, which is acting as a mass lesion. *(From Weston: Australas Radiol 13:360, 1969.)*

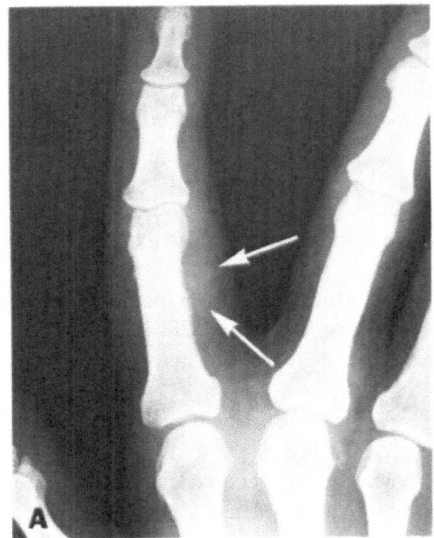
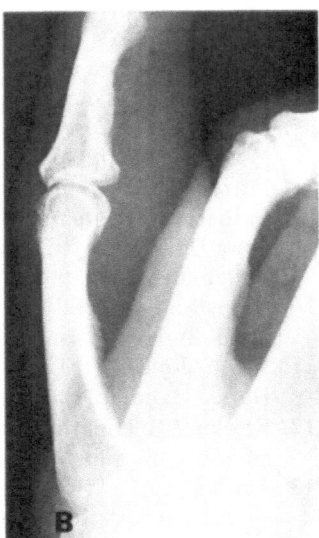
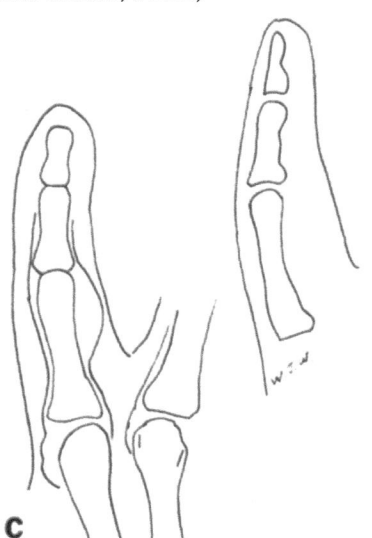

The Wrist and Hand

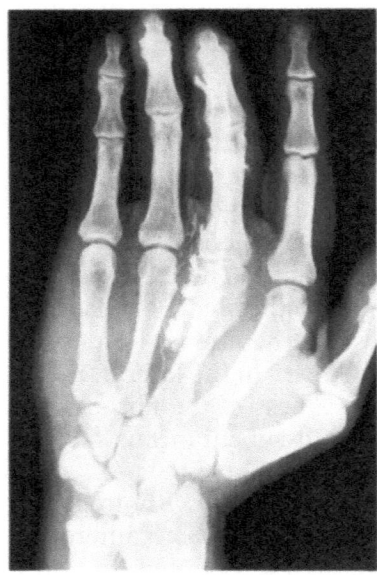

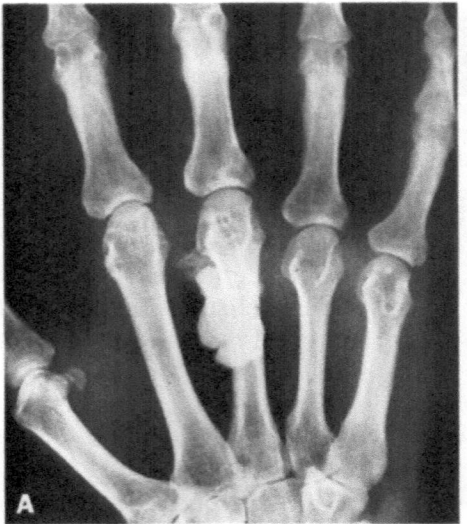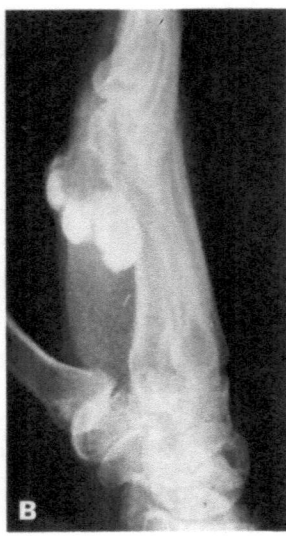

Fig. 4-37. A digital sheath involved by rheumatoid arthritis is outlined by contrast. Nodular hypertrophic synovial membrane is demonstrated and there is lymphatic filling as well. (*From Brewerton: Br J Radiol 42:487, 1969.*)

Fig. 4-38. Occasionally, in rheumatoid arthritis the proximal ends of the digital sheaths may become sacculated with extensions that pass through the palmar fascia into the subcutaneous tissues. (*From Palmer: NZ Med J 78:166, 1973.*) **A** is postero-anterior view. **B** is lateral view.

References

1. Anson BJ, Maddock WG: Callander's Surgical Anatomy, 4th ed. Philadelphia, Saunders, 1958, pp 863, 899–903
2. Backdahl M: The caput ulnae syndrome in rheumatoid arthritis. Acta Rheumatol Scand (Suppl) 5:1, 1963
3. Berens DL, Lockie LM, Lin R, et al: Roentgen changes in early rheumatoid arthritis. Radiology 82:645, 1964
4. Bourns HK, Senerkin NG: Mucoid lesions (mucoid cysts) of the fingers and toes. Clinical features and pathogenesis. Br J Surg 50:860, 1963
5. Brewerton DA: Radiographic changes in the rheumatoid hand. Br J Radiol 42:487, 1969
6. Burman M: Stenosing tendovaginitis of the dorsal and volar compartments of the wrist. Arch Surg 65:752, 1952
7. Flatt AE: The Care of the Rheumatoid Hand, 2nd ed. St. Louis, Mosby, 1968, pp 46–53
8. Frazer JE: Buchanan's Manual of Anatomy, 6th ed. London, Balliere, 1937, pp 490–492
9. Gray H: Anatomy, Descriptive and Surgical, 12th ed. London, Longmans, 1890, p 491
10. Johnston TB, Whillis J: Gray's Anatomy, Descriptive and Applied, 29th ed. London, Longmans, 1946, pp 628–630
11. Wood Jones, F: The Principles of Anatomy as Seen in the Hand. London, Balliere, 1941
12. Kaplan EB: Functional and Surgical Anatomy of the Hand. Philadelphia, Lippincott, 1953, pp 113–114
13. Kittleson AC, Whitehouse WM: Stress, greenstick, and impaction fractures. Radiol Clin North Am 4(2):281, 1966

14. Kleinert HE, Kutz JE, Fishman JH, et al: Etiology and treatment of so-called mucous cysts of the finger. J Bone Joint Surg [Am] 54:1455, 1972

15. Lewis OJ: The development of the human wrist joint during the foetal period. Anat Rec 166:499, 1971

16. Lewis OJ, Hamshere RJ, Bucknill TM: The anatomy of the wrist joint. J Anat 106:539, 1970

17. Lewis RW: The Joints of the Extremities. Springfield, Ill, Thomas, 1955, pp 27-44

18. Lockie LM: Treatment of common forms of arthritis. Ariz Med, 10:221, 1953

19. MacEwan DW: Changes due to trauma in the fat plane overlying pronator quadratus muscle. A radiological sign. Radiology 82:879, 1964

20. Martel W: The pattern of rheumatoid arthritis in the hand and wrist. Radiol Clin North Am 2(2):221, 1964

21. Martel W, Hayes JT, Duff IF: The pattern of bone erosions in the hand and wrist in rheumatoid arthritis. Radiology 84:204, 1965

22. Norrell HG: Roentgenological visualisation of the extracapsular fat. Its importance in the diagnosis of traumatic injuries to the elbow. Acta Radiol (Stockh) 42:205, 1954

23. de Quervain F: Cited by Lewis (15).

24. Ranawat CS, Straub LR: Volar tenosynovitis of the wrist in rheumatoid arthritis. Arthritis Rheum 13:112, 1970

25. Resnick D: Osteomyelitis and septic arthritis complicating hand injuries and infections. Pathogenesis of roentgenographic abnormalities. J Can Assoc Radiol 27:21, 1976

26. Resnick D: Interrelationships between radiocarpal and metacarpophalangeal joint deformities in rheumatoid arthritis. J Can Assoc Radiol 27:29, 1976

27. Resnick D: Arthrography in the evaluation of arthritic disorders of the wrist. Anatomic and pathologic considerations. Radiology 113:331, 1974

28. Resnick D: Rheumatoid arthritis of the wrist. Why the ulnar styloid? Radiology 112:29, 1974

29. Resnick D: Roentgenographic anatomy of tendon sheaths of hands and wrists. Am J Roentgenol 124:44, 1975

30. Robinson A: Cunningham's Manual of Anatomy, Vol. 1, 5th ed. Edinburgh, Frowde, 1912, p 158

31. Salter RB: Textbook of Disorders and Injuries of the Muscoloskeletal system. Baltimore, Williams & Wilkins, 1970, p 377

32. Scheldrup EW: Tendon sheath patterns in the hand. Mod Med 20:92, 1952

33. Soila P: Roentgen manifestations of adult rheumatoid arthritis. Acta Rheumatol Scand (Suppl) 1:1, 1958

34. Testut L, Jacob O: Tratto di Anatomia Topografico, 7th ed. Torino, Unione Topografica, 1943, pp. 838-841

35. Weinstein AS: Rheumatoid Arthritis of the Hand and Wrist. Veteran Administration Hospital, Cincinnati, Ohio

36. Weston WJ: De Quervain's disease. Br J Radiol 40:446, 1967

37. Weston WJ: The soft tissue changes at the wrist in rheumatoid arthritis. Australas Radiol 12:384, 1968

38. Weston WJ: The digital sheaths of the hand. Australas Radiol 13:360, 1969

39. Weston WJ: The normal arthrograms of the metacarpophalangeal, metatarsophalangeal and interphalangeal joints. Australas Radiol 13:211, 1969
40. Weston WJ: Joint space widening with intracapsular fractures in joints of the fingers and toes of children. Australas Radiol 15:367, 1971
41. Weston WJ: The soft tissue signs of the enlarged ulnar bursa in rheumatoid arthritis. J Can Assoc Radiol 24:282, 1973
42. Weston WJ: The ulnar bursa. Australas Radiol 17:216, 1973
43. Weston WJ, Kelsey CK: Functional anatomy of the pisicuneiform joint. Br J Radiol 46:692, 1973

CHAPTER 5

The Hip

RADIOLOGIC ANATOMY OF THE HIP JOINT AND ASSOCIATED BURSAE

Arthrography of the hip joint performed on the cadaver may be undertaken to demonstrate the normal appearance of the synovial membrane about the hip joint. The average hip joint will take about 12 ml of contrast medium (Fig. 5-1). The contrast medium is seen in the arthrogram as a thin layer above the femoral head. The ligamentum teres may be seen on the medial aspect of the head encircled by contrast medium. The ligamentum transversum spans the cotyloid notch making an indentation in the contrast medium below the ligamentum teres.

The orbicular ligament produces a waist above and below the femoral neck. On the under surface of the neck the inferior articular recess is seen medially, and the recessus coli is seen laterally above and below the femoral neck. The supraarticular recess lies above the limbus (4,7,8). In one case at postmortem the hip was overdistended with 25 ml of contrast medium. The impression of the orbicular ligament was then well seen, as was the bulging synovial membrane on the caudal aspect of the neck, medial and lateral to the orbicular ligament (Fig. 5-2A and B).

The principal bursae in the region are those deep to gluteus medius and minimus. The bursa deep to gluteus minimus

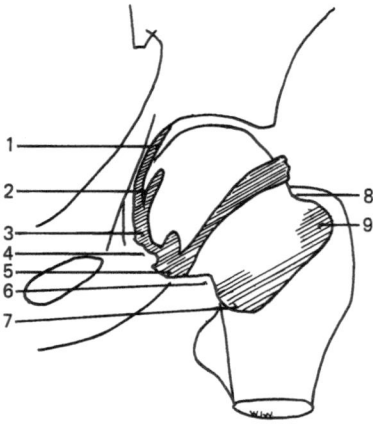

Fig. 5-1. Line diagram of postmortem arthrogram of hip following injection of 12 ml of barium suspension. 1, recessus capitis; 2, ligamentum teres; 3, acetabular recess; 4, ligamentum transversum; 5, inferior recess; 6 and 8, zona orbicularis; 7 and 9, recessus coli. (*From Weston: Acta Radiol (Diagn) 10:326, 1970.*)

lies anteromedially to that of gluteus medius, on the anterior aspect of the upper portion of the greater trochanter. This bursa is approached from the anterolateral aspect of the greater trochanter. A scalp vein needle can be used in a thin subject at postmortem examination. The tip of the needle must touch the anterior aspect of the greater trochanter. A small volume of barium sulfate (0.25 ml) is sufficient to outline the bursa (Fig. 5-3).

The bursa deep to gluteus medius is approached from the lateral aspect of the greater trochanter. The scalp vein needle must have its tip touching bone. The capacity at this bursa varies from 0.5 to 3 ml (Fig. 5-4) (13).

In Figure 5-4 the extrasynovial fat is well shown between the bursa and the bone. This is a feature of all bursae which have been studied. A further significant feature is shown in Figure 5-5, where the bursa deep to gluteus medius has been filled and an arthrogram of the hip performed at the same time. This figure demonstrates that gluteus medius is some distance from the capsule of the hip joint, and thus it is impossible for that muscle and the extramuscular fat lying deep to it to be displaced by a hip joint effusion.

SOFT TISSUE CHANGES

Hefke and Turner (5) discussed the obturator sign in diagnosis of septic arthritis and tuberculosis of the hip joint. This was seen as a swelling of the obturator internus on the lateral wall of the pelvis in the anteroposterior view. It was later reported by Drey (3) that synovitis of the hip joint produced

Fig. 5-2. Postmortem arthrogram using 25 ml of barium sulfate suspension. **A.** Anteroposterior view. **B.** AP view with lower limb abducted and externally rotated. The inferior recess is well seen caudal to the femoral neck. (*From Weston: Acta Radiol (Diagn) 10:326, 1970.*)

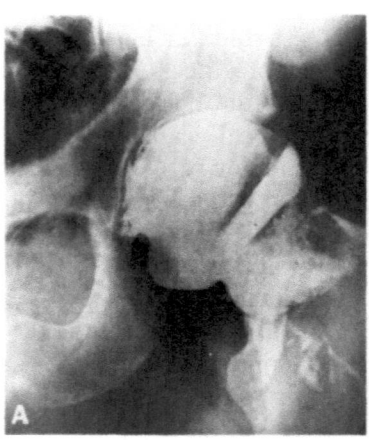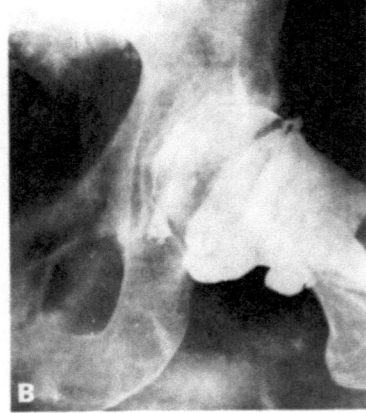

Soft Tissues of the Extremities

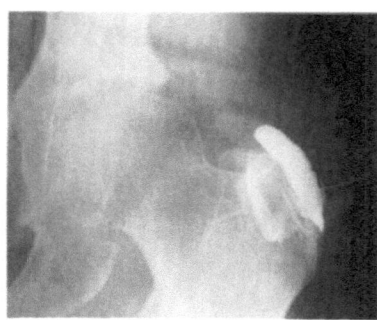

Fig. 5-3. The bursa deep to gluteus minimus lies anteromedial to that of gluteus medius. Both bursae are intimately related to the greater trochanter. (*From Weston: Australas Radiol 14:325, 1970.*)

Fig. 5-4. The bursa deep to gluteus medius is larger than that deep to gluteus minimus (Fig. 5-3). It extends up above the greater trochanter. The extrasynovial fat is well seen between the barium-filled bursa and bone. (*From Weston: Australas Radiol 14:325, 1970.*)

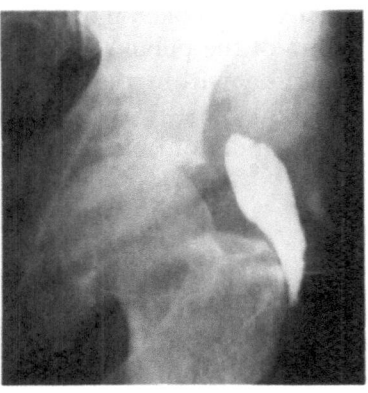

swelling both of gluteus minimus, the most medial of the gluteal muscles lying above and lateral to the joint, and of iliopsoas just above its insertion to the lesser trochanter, below and medial to the joint.

Kellgren (6) stated that "the clinical diagnosis of early hip joint involvement in rheumatoid arthritis is difficult because pain in the leg is so easily attributed to the more obvious concurrent disease in the knees, and the small effusions in the hips are not easily demonstrated." Cartilage loss and the wedge-shaped appearance of the superior part of the joint space are well-known later signs of rheumatoid involvement of the hip.

Berens (1) drew attention to such soft tissue signs as capsular swelling and synovial involvement in the early stage of hip joint involvement in rheumatoid arthritis. Sosman (10) also mentioned the capsular contour as seen against the fat pad above the hip, ie, between the superior acetabular margin and the greater trochanter, and, as is especially well seen in children, the fat and muscle line which is visible inferiorly. Reichmann (9) stated that it is impossible to identify the upper capsular contour with certainty.

Brown (2) has investigated the capsular fat pad above the hip. He noted that it moved laterally when the hip was abducted and externally rotated, or abducted and internally rotated. Medial rotation brought the fat pad closer to the femoral neck. Dissection showed that this fatty layer lies anterior to the femoral neck.

In our experience the distended joint capsule caudal to the joint, produced by the rheumatoid synovial mass lesion, can be demonstrated radiographically in the axial view of the hip when the soft tissues are cleared from bone (12).

In a child the pattern of synovial effusions is different from the pattern seen in the adult. With an effusion in the hip joint of a child there is initially an increase in the width of the joint space between the femoral head and the medial acetabular wall. The "frog" view of the hip demonstrates that the whole of the joint space is wider than the normal uninvolved side. A pair of calipers is necessary to measure this joint space widening. It is imperative to have the lower limbs in a symmetric position when these measurements are made. A transient synovitis (irritable hip syndrome) produces no more than this joint space widening. With a septic arthritis, joint space widening is accompanied by edema of the surrounding tissues which obliterates the fatty planes in Scarpa's triangle. As the septic arthritis settles the edema in Scarpa's triangle diminishes.

The other radiologic appearances are of no diagnostic value. The obturator sign can be seen in normal hips and is only evidence that the pelvis is asymmetric. The displacement of the fat pad cephalic to the femoral neck can also be

The Hip

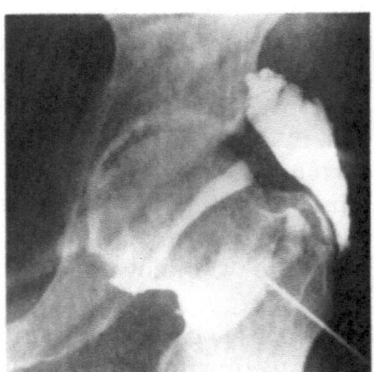

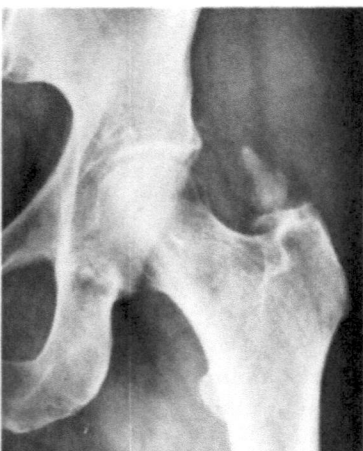

Fig. 5-5. An arthrogram has been performed on the hip following the outlining of the bursa deep to gluteus medius. Both gluteus medius and the fat deep to it are remote from the hip joint. (*From Weston: Australas Radiol 14:325, 1970.*)

Fig. 5-6. A large area of calcification is noted in the trochanteric area. This is a tendinitis calcarea.

varied by the position of the limb and, in accord with Reichmann (9), is of no value as a soft tissue sign. This same author considered that body build and the degree of muscular contraction could also alter the appearances. Brown (2) commented that with a transient synovitis the limb is internally rotated and abducted, and thus one would expect to see the capsular fat pad displaced laterally. This is in fact what is seen.

Tendinitis Calcarea

Fig. 5-7. A further area of calcification lies in the gluteal region and is of different shape than that seen in Figure 5-6.

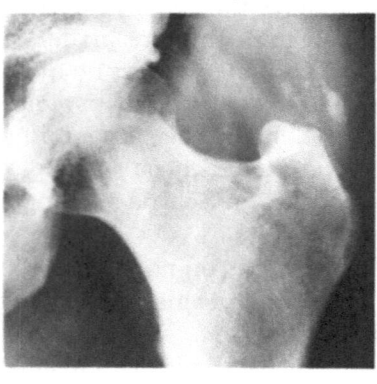

Tendinitis calcarea is occasionally associated with pain in the region of the hip. The calcification commonly lies in the gluteal insertions into the greater trochanter. This area is often overexposed on films and can be easily overlooked if a search of this area is not made in every film of the pelvis (Figs. 5-6 and 5-7). No examples of calcification within the gluteal bursae have been found but one could expect to see this on rare occasions since it is seen in the subdeltoid bursa at the shoulder.

Osteochondromatosis

Synovial osteochondromatosis is a rare finding in the hip. However, it is important to consider the pattern of this disease process, which should be sought as a cause of otherwise

Soft Tissues of the Extremities

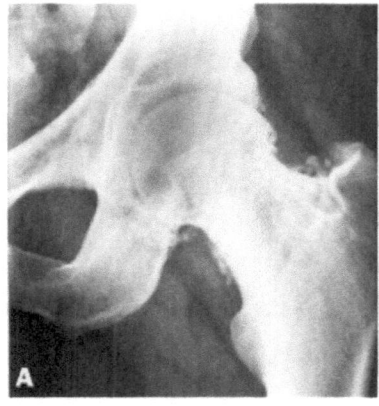

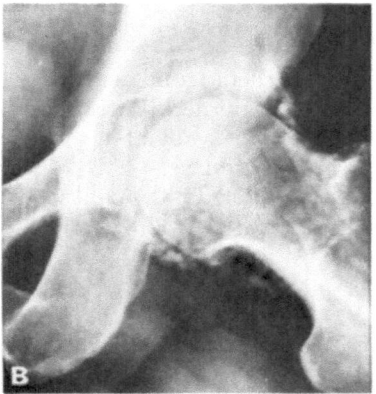

Fig. 5-8. Osteochondromatosis of the hip joint. The bony masses are seen where there is synovial membrane. The anatomy determines the radiographic appearance. **A.** Anteroposterior view. **B.** Anteroposterior view with lower limb abducted and externally rotated.

unexplained chronic hip pain. One can expect to see the osteochondromatous masses wherever there is synovial membrane and the pattern is governed by the anatomy of the synovium. It is easier to identify the lesions caudal to the femoral neck (Fig. 5-8).

The Pectoneal Bursa

The pectoneal bursa (iliopsoas bursa) is bounded anteriorly by the iliopsoas, laterally by the iliofemoral ligament, medially by the cotyloid ligament, and posteriorly by the pectoneal eminence and the thin part of the hip joint capsule. Poupart's ligament lies above while the pubofemoral ligament lies below it. According to Staple (11) the bursa communicates with the hip joint in 15 percent of cases.

When the bursa is enlarged, it appears as a mass in the groin that is fixed, nontender, and nonpulsatile, and which lies below the lateral half of Poupart's ligament. It may extend under the inguinal ligament into the retroperitoneal area and displace cecum, ureter, or bladder. Rheumatoid arthritis or degenerative joint disease may lead to enlargement of the bursa, especially when it communicates with the hip joint. Villonodular synovitis can also affect the bursa. Bursography may aid in the diagnosis and if the bursa communicates with the hip joint the bursa may be demonstrated by arthrography.

RHEUMATOID DISEASE

Study of the normal arthrogram demonstrates that the main synovial bulk lies below the femoral neck. The synovial

Fig. 5-9. Anteroposterior **(A)** and axial **(B)** roentgenograms in a case of active rheumatoid arthritis. The synovial mass lesion is well seen caudal to the femoral neck in the axial view (arrow). Erosions and cartilage loss are also noted. (*From Weston: Acta Radiol (Diagn) 10:326, 1970.*)

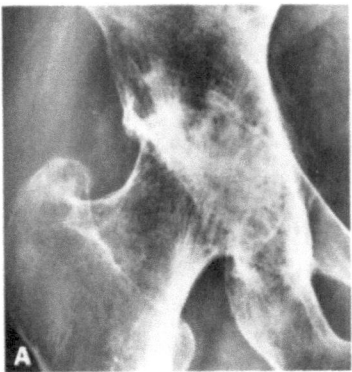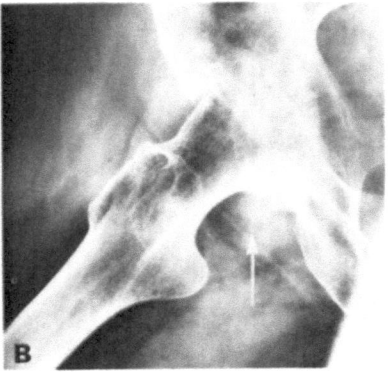

The Hip

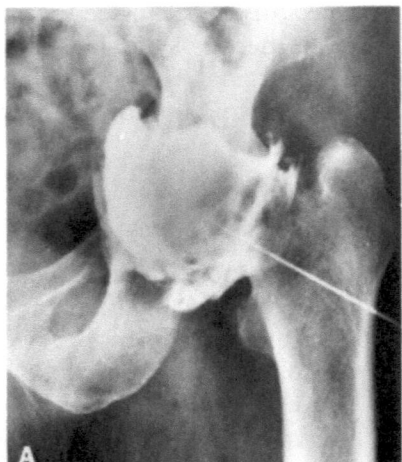 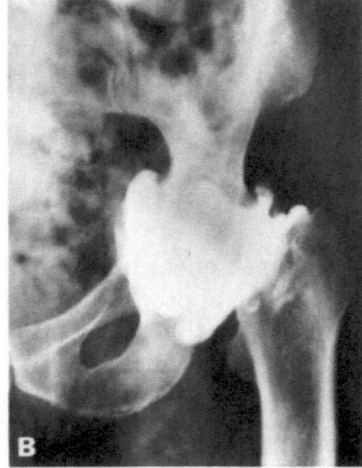 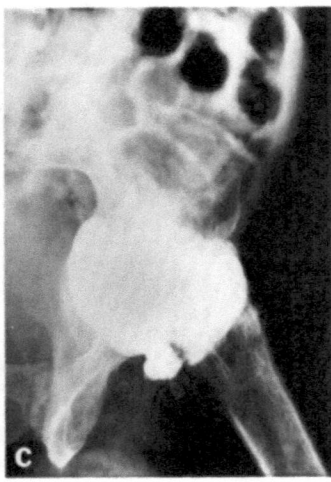

Fig. 5-10. Arthrograms in a case of active rheumatoid arthritis. Distended capsular recess caudal to the femoral neck, associated with nodular filling defects of the hypertrophic synovial membrane. **A.** Anteroposterior view in filling phase. **B.** Anteroposterior view with injection completed. **C.** Axial view with injection completed. (*From Weston: Acta Radiol (Diagn) 10:326, 1970.*)

swelling in rheumatoid arthritis produces a mass lesion on the under surface of the femoral neck. The soft tissue mass lesion in the standard anteroposterior film can be hidden by the overlying ischiopubic ramus. The overlying bones are cleared in the axial view, in which the caudal soft tissue changes are seen to their best advantage (Fig. 5-9) (12). The

Fig. 5-11. Arthrograms in a further case of active rheumatoid arthritis. Distended capsular recess caudal to femoral neck. Note filling of lymphatic vessels. **A.** Anteroposterior view in filling phase. **B.** Anteroposterior view with injection completed. **C.** Axial view with injection completed. (*From Weston: Acta Radiol (Diagn) 10:326, 1970.*)

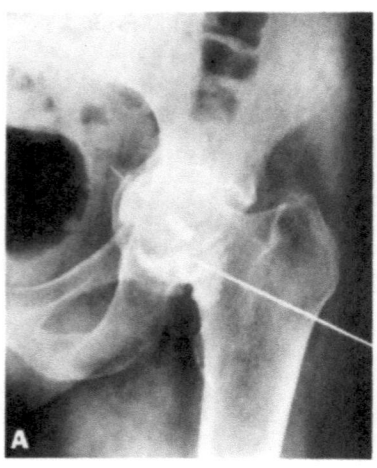 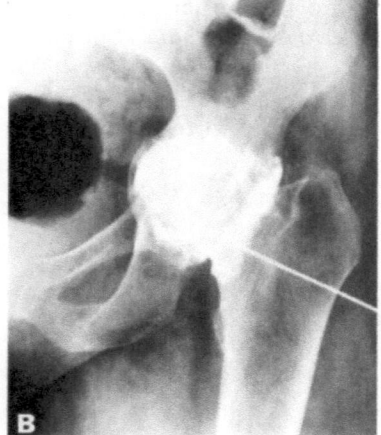 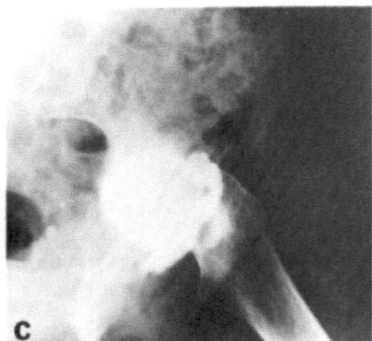

Soft Tissues of the Extremities

soft tissues cephalic to the femoral neck are difficult to assess, as there is considerable variation in this area depending on the position of the limb.

Arthrograms in two cases with rheumatoid arthritis of the hips are shown in Figures 5-10 and 5-11. The widest portion of the joint recesses may be seen caudal to the femoral neck. Rheumatoid arthritis produces an enlargement of the capsular recesses, as demonstrated by Weston (12). The hypertrophic synovial membrane with its nodular filling defects is well seen in these arthrograms. In one of these cases (Fig. 5-11) there was filling of the lymphatics about the hip joint, which is further evidence of the rheumatoid process.

References

1. Berens DL: Hips. In: Carter Mary E(ed): Radiological Aspects of Rheumatoid Arthritis. International Congress Series No. 61. Amsterdam, Excerpta Medica, 1963, p 307
2. Brown I: A study of the "capsular" shadow in disorders of the hip in children. J Bone Joint Surg [Br] 57:175, 1975
3. Drey L: A roentgenographic study of transitory synovitis of the hip joint. Radiology 60:588, 1953
4. Fischer FK: Joint injuries. Arthrography. In Schinz HR, Baensch WE, Friedl E, et al (eds): Roentgen Diagnosis, Vol. 2. New York, Grune & Stratton, 1952, p. 1218
5. Hefke HW, Turner VC: The obturator sign as the earliest roentgenographic sign in diagnosis of septic arthritis and tuberculosis of the hip. Br. J Bone Joint Surg 24:857, 1942
6. Kellgren JH: The hip joint. In Carter Mary E (ed): Radiological Aspects of Rheumatoid Arthritis. International Congress Series No. 61. Amsterdam, Excerpta Medica, 1963, p 301
7. Lindblom K: Arthrography. In McLaren JW (ed): Modern Trends in Diagnostic Radiology, 2nd Series. London, Butterworth, 1953, p 251
8. Lindblom K: Arthrography. J Faculty Radiol 3:151, 1952
9. Reichmann S: Roentgenologic soft tissue appearances in hip joint disease. Acta Radiol [Diagn] (Stockh) 6:167, 1967
10. Sosman JL: Hips. In Carter Mary E (ed) Radiological Aspects of Rheumatoid Arthritis. International Congress Series No. 61, Amsterdam, Excerpta Medica, 1963, p 307
11. Staple TW: Arthrographic demonstration of the iliopsoas bursa extension of the hip joint. Radiology 102:515, 1972
12. Weston WJ: Synovial lesions in the adult hip joint in rheumatoid arthritis. Acta Radiol (Diagn) 10:326, 1970
13. Weston WJ: The bursa deep to gluteus medius and minimus. Australas Radiol 14:325, 1970

CHAPTER 6

The Knee

RADIOLOGIC ANATOMY

Balazs et al (1) noted that the normal knee joint contains 5 to 8 ml of synovial fluid. This is the only normal joint in which fluid can be recognized radiographically. In the suprapatellar area this fluid can be seen in the lateral x-ray as a rectangular opacity running upward and forward from the edge of the articular surface of the femoral condyle (Fig. 6-1). There is a triangular mass of extrasynovial fat between the fluid and the quadriceps tendon cephalic to the patella. The suprapatellar pouch continues up on to the posterior aspect of the quadriceps and cannot be separated from it. Posterior to the synovial fluid, a further mass of fat lies ventral to the femur. Fluid may also be seen between the femoral condyles and the upper surface of the infrapatellar pad of fat. The layer of fluid here becomes continuous with that between the under surface of the triangular pad and the smooth upper surface of the tibia ventral to the tibial spine. This layer of fluid is 1 to 2 mm in thickness. In the anteroposterior view of the knee, the fluid lies medially and laterally to the joint margins of the tibia and femur. The medial and lateral ligaments form a clear-cut boundary to this fluid. The medial and lateral boundaries of the distended suprapatellar pouch are seen as curved lines which are convex in relation to the medial and lateral aspects of the femur. These changes have been well described by Harris and Hecht (6) and have been reproduced

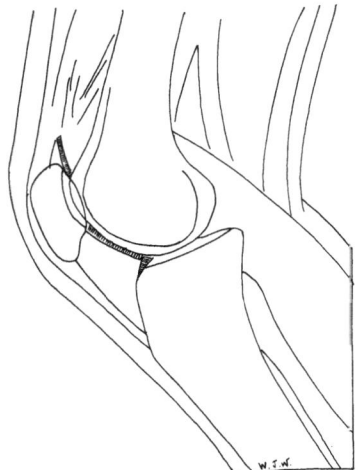

Fig. 6-1. Line diagram showing the normal synovial fluid in the suprapatellar pouch (hatched area). This fluid becomes continuous with that above and below the triangular pad of fat.

Fig. 6-2. The deep infrapatellar bursa has been outlined by contrast medium. It lies in intimate contact with the tibia cephalic to the tibial tuberosity. (*From Weston: Australas Radiol 17:212, 1973.*)

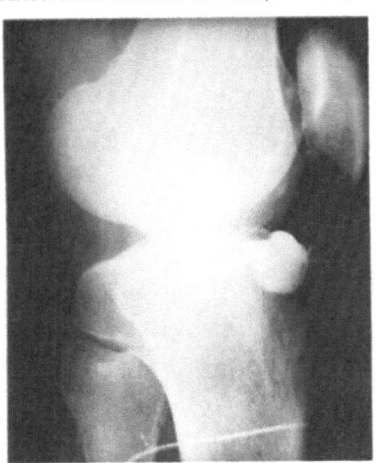

by postmortem injection of water followed by contrast media. Lewis's book on the extremities (11) should be consulted by all those interested in earlier descriptions of the suprapatellar pouch.

Anterior to the infrapatellar pad of fat is the infrapatellar ligament, which is clearly defined in the lateral view as a homogeneous structure about 5 mm in thickness. The deep infrapatellar bursa is a potential space and lies between the ligamentum patellae and the smooth ventral aspect of the tibia proximal to the tibial tuberosity. The bursa can be outlined by contrast media injected into it percutaneously (Fig. 6-2). The tip of the butterfly needle is introduced percutaneously cephalic to the tibial tuberosity until it strikes bone. Contrast medium (0.25 to 0.5 ml) is injected to outline the bursa which, when enlarged, can act as a space-taking lesion within the triangular infrapatellar pad of fat.

The extrasynovial and capsular fat pads on the posterior aspect of the knee joint are important landmarks. Lewis (11) and Berens and Lin (3) have noted that the fatty translucencies behind the knee joint may be displaced backward by effusions. The detailed anatomy of the fat pads on the posterior aspect of the knee has been described and a further sign of effusion in the knee—fabella displacement—noted (18,19). In the lateral film of the knee, a thin layer of extrasynovial fat is visible following the posterior curve of the femoral condyles. This terminates proximally just above the origin of the condyle, while below it unites with a similar fatty layer on the posterior aspect of the lateral tibial condyle. This configuration forms the so-called synovial bird, a numeral 3–shaped double curve. The inferior fat pad overlies the synovial cavity where it surrounds the popliteus tendon and extends about 1.5 cm below the tibial plateau. The relationship of these fat pads to the synovial joint space can be demonstrated by arthrography (Fig. 6-3).

The cruciate ligaments are covered by synovial membrane on their anterior, lateral, and medial aspects, but not posteriorly. Here, the posterior cruciate ligament is outlined above by fat, which may be visible in the lateral view of the knee (Fig. 6-4A and B). Behind this fat is a condensation of the posterior capsule of the knee joint, and this in turn has a fat pad between it and the inner and outer bellies of gastrocnemius. Thus, the joint capsule in the midline may be made visible by fat and may be seen just posterior to the junction of the two parts of the numeral 3–shaped translucency (Fig. 6-5A and B). The surrounding capsular fat pads are best seen in infants. The outer head of gastrocnemius arises from just above the femoral condyle and from the posterior aspect of the capsule of the knee joint. Thus, a fabella, when present, lies in the capsule, its deep surface articulating with the lateral condyle of the femur (7).

The Knee

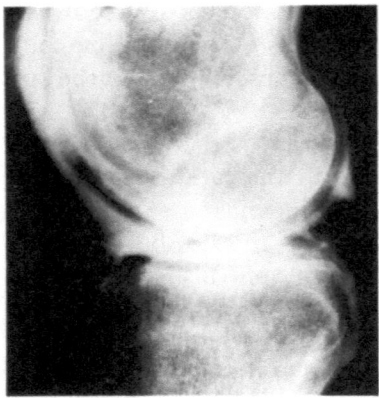

Fig. 6-3. Lateral view of a knee arthrogram. The opaque medium posteriorly outlines the double curve which appears as a numeral 3 in this view.

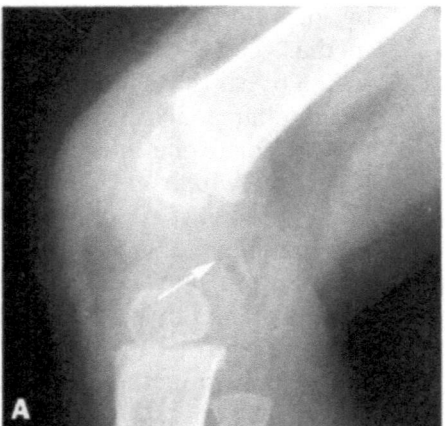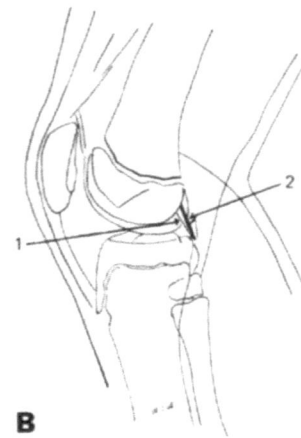

Fig. 6-4. A. Lateral view of a knee of an infant showing a pad of fat cephalic and dorsal to the posterior cruciate ligament (arrow). Both structures pass upward and forward. **B.** Line diagram of **A**. 1, posterior cruciate ligament; 2, thickened capsule posteriorly. (*From Weston: Br J Radiol 44:277, 1971.*)

Arthrography of the normal knee joint is performed with the patient lying supine and the quadriceps relaxed. The patella is displaced laterally by the left hand of the operator and a needle is introduced through the skin fat and capsule until it tips the under surface of the patella. Twelve ml of contrast media is injected into the knee joint to demonstrate the synovial cavity. The contrast outlines the suprapatellar pouch which extends up 7 to 10 cm from the joint line. The contrast

Fig. 6-5. A. Lateral radiograph showing the vertical linear opacity posteriorly, produced by the thickened capsule in the knee joint of an adult (arrow). A fat pad lies between the capsule and the heads of the gastrocnemius posteriorly. **B.** Line diagram of **A**, showing the relationship of the extrasynovial fat pads (stippled) to those of the posterior joint capsule. (*From Weston: Br J Radiol 44:277, 1971.*)

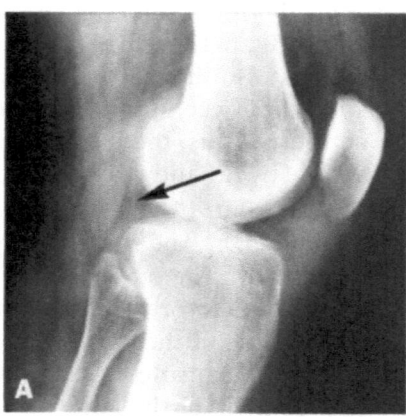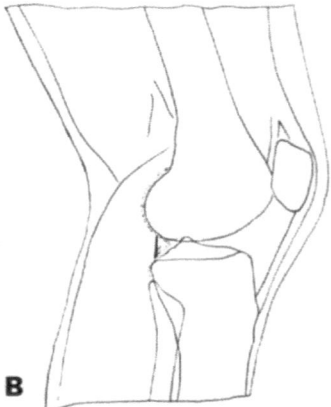

Soft Tissues of the Extremities

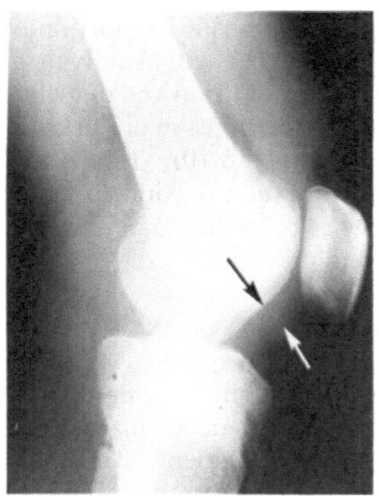

Fig. 6-6. A large effusion is seen in the suprapatellar pouch outlined by extrasynovial fat. The effusion (arrows) separates the femoral condyles from the infrapatellar pad of fat. It extends to separate the upper surface of the tibia from the under surface of the pad of fat.

Fig. 6-7. With a large effusion in the knee joint the patella and the ligamentum patellae are displaced forward.

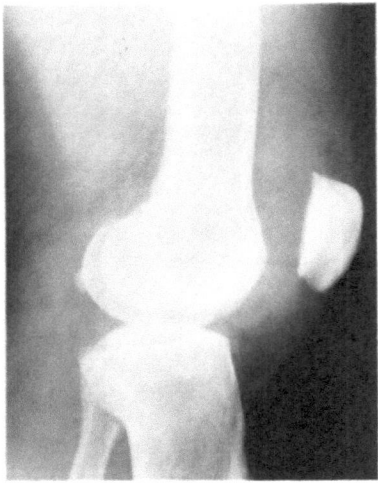

extends over the femoral condyles and the upper surface of the infrapatellar pad of fat. Further extension occurs between the under surface of the infrapatellar fat pad and the smooth ventral surface of the upper end of the tibia, cephalic to the tibial tuberosity. The pattern substantiates the soft tissue findings in the lateral view of the knee. In the anteroposterior projection of the normal arthrogram contrast medium is noted in the suprapatellar pouch on the medial aspect of the lower end of the femur. To a lesser extent, the contrast can be seen in the pouch on the lateral aspect of the femur. At the joint line, contrast can be seen between the internal and external lateral ligaments and between the femoral and tibial condyles. It extends into the medial and lateral compartments of the knee joint to outline the menisci.

SOFT TISSUE CHANGES

An effusion into the knee, be it a transudate, exudate, or hemarthrosis, produces the following changes in the lateral view. The suprapatellar pouch becomes visible and ovoid in outline with a rounded cephalic pole. The pouch is surrounded by extrasynovial fat and, as a result, is clearly defined. A large, dense collection of blood causes a more marked soft tissue change.

The fluid also separates the femoral condyles from the upper surface of the triangular infrapatellar pad of fat. The larger the effusion, the greater the downward and forward displacement of this surface (Fig. 6-6). The triangular fat pad thus loses its normal shape and becomes more trapezoidal or rectangular in outline. With large effusions the ligamentum patellae and the patella are displaced forward away from the femur and tibia (Fig. 6-7). In the anteroposterior projection the internal and external lateral ligaments are displaced away from the tibia and femur, and with large effusions the knee becomes spindle-shaped. Above the patella, the extrasynovial fat about the suprapatellar pouch may become visible on the medial aspect. This appearance has been well described by Harris and Hecht (6), who noted a curved lucent line with its convexity directed away from the medial aspect of the femur. Though a lucent line is more common on the medial than on the lateral side, a lucent line may appear on both sides of the femur in the presence of a large effusion.

In some synovial effusions of the knee joint, the extrasynovial fat pads may be displaced posteriorly into the popliteal fossa. They retain their numeral 3–shape as the effusion increases (Fig. 6-8). In patients with an ossified fabella a further sign becomes evident in the posterior component of the effusion. The fabella is displaced posteriorly by distension of the capsule in which it lies (Fig. 6-9A–C) (18). When

The Knee

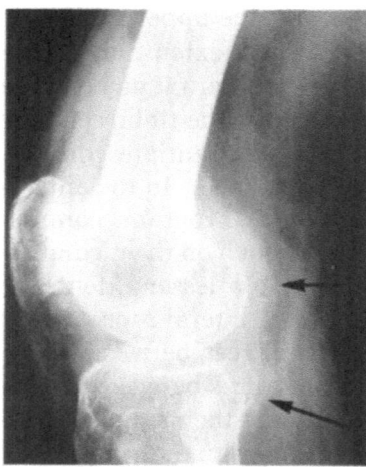

Fig. 6-8. A large synovial effusion in the knee joint, where the extrasynovial fat pads are visible and are displaced posteriorly into the popliteal fossa. They retain their numeral 3–shape as the effusion increases (arrows).

loose bodies or foreign bodies lie in the posterior portion of the joint near the lateral tibial condyle, they will usually have a convexity directed posteriorly. Their position and distribution are determined by the shape of the extension of the synovial cavity over the popliteus tendon (Fig. 6-10). This extension of the joint space is an important feature, since it is not always appreciated that opacities seen in this region can be within the synovial cavity of the joint.

The Prepatellar Bursa—Bursitis

With involvement of the prepatellar bursa, whether by trauma or infection, a space-taking homogeneous mass lesion can be seen anterior to the infrapatellar ligament. This mass displaces the cutis line forward (Fig. 6-11). Both an infected and a traumatic bursitis will produce surrounding edema which extends both cranially and caudally from the enlarged bursa. A bursitis can easily be distinguished on the soft tissue study and separated from an intraarticular effusion. Bursography has shown that the prepatellar bursa and the infrapatellar bursa may communicate (Fig. 6-12). Dystrophic calcification may be a sequel of a chronic bursitis (Fig. 6-13A and B).

Fig. 6-9. A. Lateral view of knee in a patient with psoriatic arthropathy. The fabella (arrow), which is part intracapsular, is displaced posteriorly. The posterior extrasynovial fat pads are well seen. **B.** Arthrogram of the knee (anteroposterior view) of patient with psoriatic arthropathy. The synovial prolongation about the tendon of popliteus is well shown and forms the lower half of the numeral 3. **C.** Arthrogram of the knee (lateral view). The fabella is displaced posteriorly because it is partly intracapsular in position. (*From Weston: Br J Radiol 44:277, 1971.*)

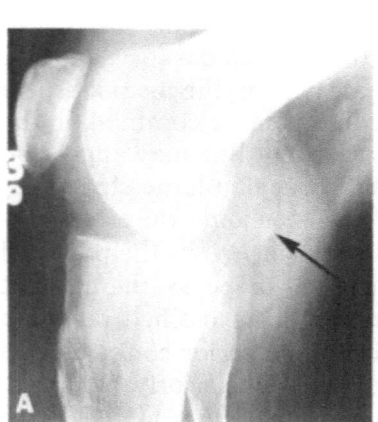
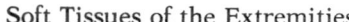
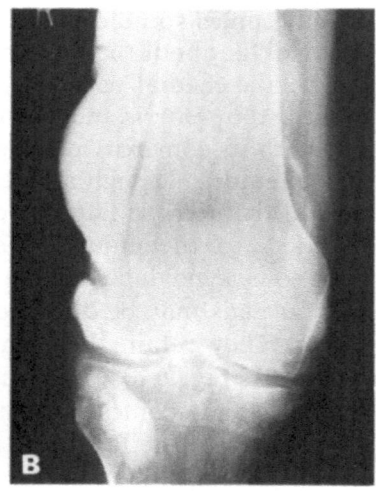
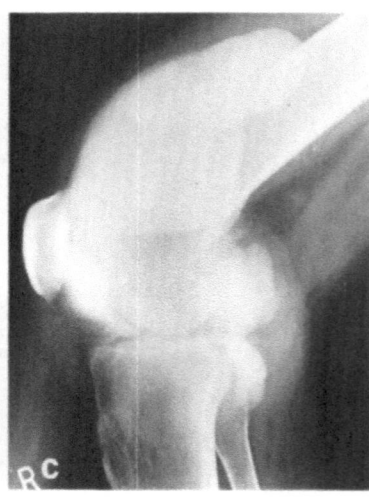

Soft Tissues of the Extremities

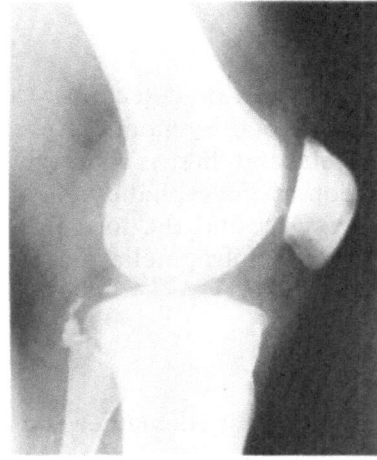

Fig. 6-10. Lateral view of the knee in a patient with osteochondritis dissecans. Several loose bodies are noted behind the lateral tibial condyle. Their position and distribution are determined by the shape of the synovial cavity about the popliteus tendon. (*From Weston: Br J Radiol 44:277, 1971.*)

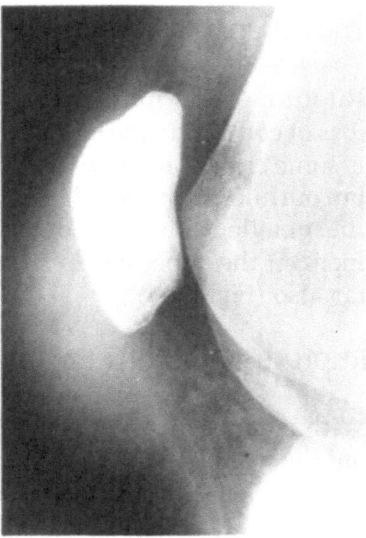

Fig. 6-11. Patient with a traumatic prepatellar bursitis. A homogeneous soft tissue mass is noted anterior to the patella and ligamentum patellae.

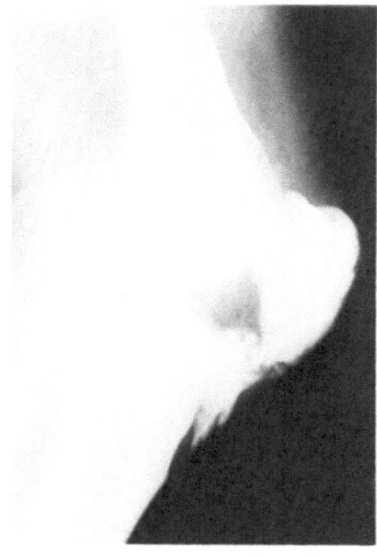

Fig. 6-12. Bursography of an enlarged prepatellar bursa shows that it communicates with the infrapatellar bursa.

Fig. 6-13. **A.** Anteroposterior view of a calcified bursa. **B.** Lateral view of **A**.

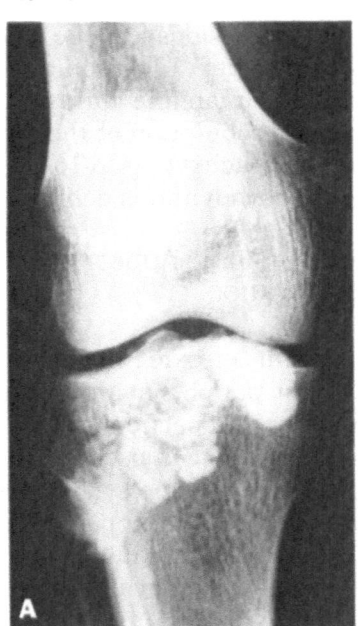

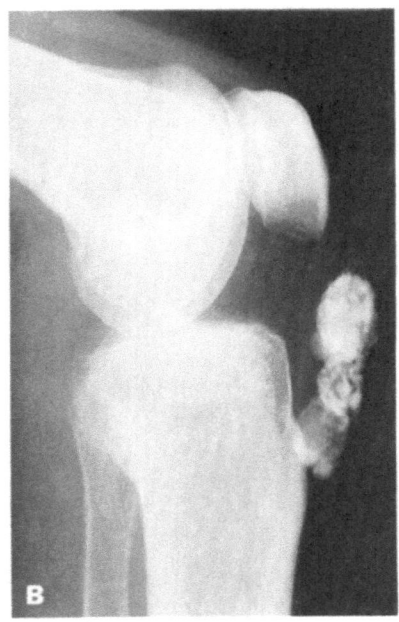

The Knee

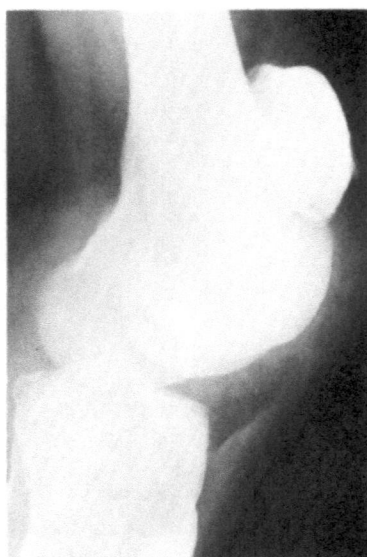

Fig. 6-14. Rupture of the ligamentum patellae is shown by a loss in continuity of that structure. The patella is displaced centrally. Marked edema is seen ventral to the site of rupture and in the infrapatellar pad of fat.

Fig. 6-15. A rupture of the quadriceps expansion above the patella. Gross edema is seen in that area. The ligamentum patellae is somewhat wavy in outline.

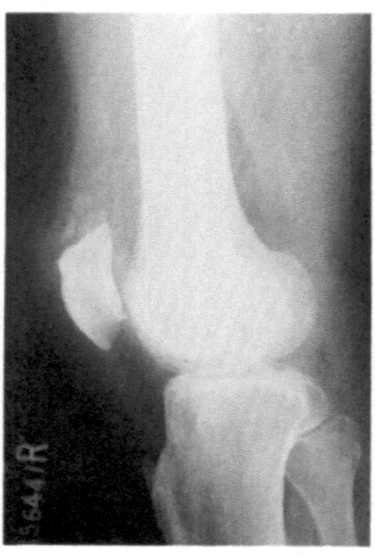

The Infrapatellar Ligament—Rupture

Rupture of the infrapatellar ligament can be detected by a loss of continuity in the soft tissue mass of this tendon. There is some cranial migration of the patella and there is an irregular outline to the quadriceps tendon at the cephalic pole of the patella. Marked edema appears around the torn ligament in the subcutaneous fat and in the infrapatellar pad of fat also (Fig. 6-14).

Rupture of the Quadriceps Tendon

With rupture of the quadriceps tendon gross edema develops on the ventral aspect of the lower thigh with loss of the normal clear definition between the subcutaneous fat and the deep fascia. Some fluid may be seen in the suprapatellar pouch. The ligamentum patellae is no longer taut and may become somewhat undulant in outline. The quadriceps tendon, which is normally convex ventrally, migrates cranially and loses its convex outline (Fig. 6-15).

Pigmented Villonodular Synovitis

Staple (15) stated that "Tumors of the synovial membrane may present as isolated masses or diffuse irregular infiltration of the synovium. Pigmented villonodular synovitis is the most common synovial tumor and may be present in either a solitary nodular or diffuse form." There may be no associated bone or cartilage abnormality and soft tissue calcification may be absent. It is essential to have good soft tissue detail and the use of industrial film is desirable (10).

These lesions can be demonstrated by double contrast arthrography. The solitary nodular lesion is easier to demonstrate than the diffuse form. The latter will show increased lobulation of the synovial membrane and decreased joint capacity (Fig. 6-16A). The vascular nature of the involved synovium is demonstrated in Figure 6-16B.

Radiographic Appearance of Osmium in the Soft Tissues of the Knee

Osmium tetroxide has been used as an intraarticular injection in patients with rheumatoid arthritis of the knee, in Scandinavia particularly. Ten ml of the 1 percent solution of this chemical is used for this procedure. It leaves a dark black stain in the synovial membrane which is apparent at synovectomy. Preoperative radiographs show a dense opacity in the suprapatellar pouch (20). Osmium has an atomic number of 76 (bariums atomic number is 56). Radiographs of the excised membrane demonstrate a metallic density on

Soft Tissues of the Extremities

Fig. 6-16. A. Arthrogram of the knee (lateral view). A diffuse nodular mass lesion is noted in the suprapatellar pouch. It was shown to be a pigmented villonodular synovitis. **B.** An arteriogram in the arterial phase in the same patient showing increased vascularity to the tumor mass.

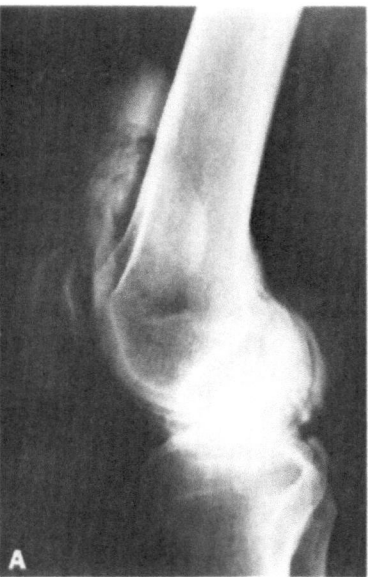
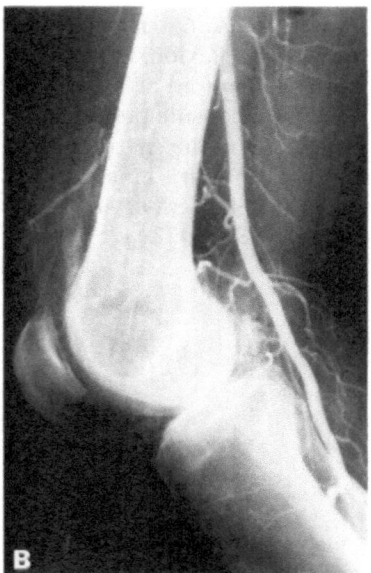

the film that corresponds to the reduced black osmium seen on the excised synovium.

RHEUMATOID DISEASE

With involvement of the synovial membrane of the knee joint in the rheumatoid process, edema, synovial hypertrophy, synovitis, and rice-grain bodies may all contribute to the soft tissue mass. In the active phase, synovial changes are very commonly seen between the deep surface of the infrapatellar pad of fat and that part of the tibia lying anterior to the tibial spine. The presence of synovial tissue here explains why this is a common site for erosions seen on radiographs and at operation.

In the active phase of rheumatoid disease the enlargement of the synovial cavity can be demonstrated by arthrography (17). Synovial hypertrophy produces space-taking nodular masses which are fixed when viewed under a television screen, in contrast to mobile, loose bodies. The rice-grain bodies and the synovial hypertrophy are best seen in the early filling phase of the arthrogram. Lymphatic filling has already been referred to as one of the features of the arthrogram in rheumatoid arthritis, and this is seen at the knee. Examples have been noted in published figures such as that in a paper by Taylor (16), although the phenomenon has not received comment. Synovial hypertrophy, edema, and effusion may also produce an irregular mass posteriorly. In the case shown in Figure 6-17, the mass has displaced the calcified popliteal artery posteriorly. These posterior synovial masses are very common in the rheumatic group of diseases.

Fig. 6-17. A patient with rheumatoid arthritis of the right knee of 4 years' duration. An irregular synovial mass is noted on the posterior aspect of the knee joint (arrow). It displaces the calcified popliteal artery posteriorly. The synovial mass also involves the suprapatellar pouch above and the infrapatellar fat pad below. (*From Weston: Br J Radiol 44:277, 1971.*)

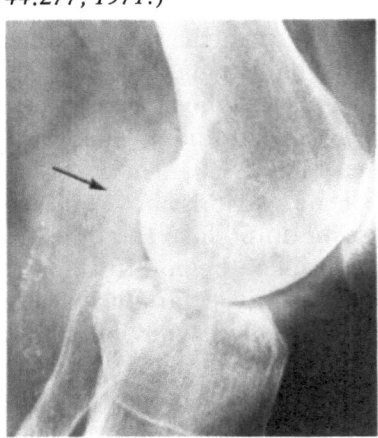

The Knee

Fig. 6-18. A. Lateral view of the knee in flexion, in a patient with rheumatoid arthritis. The thickened capsule posteriorly has taken on the shape of a numeral 3. **B.** Line diagram of **A.** (*From Weston: Australas Radiol 16:89, 1972.*)

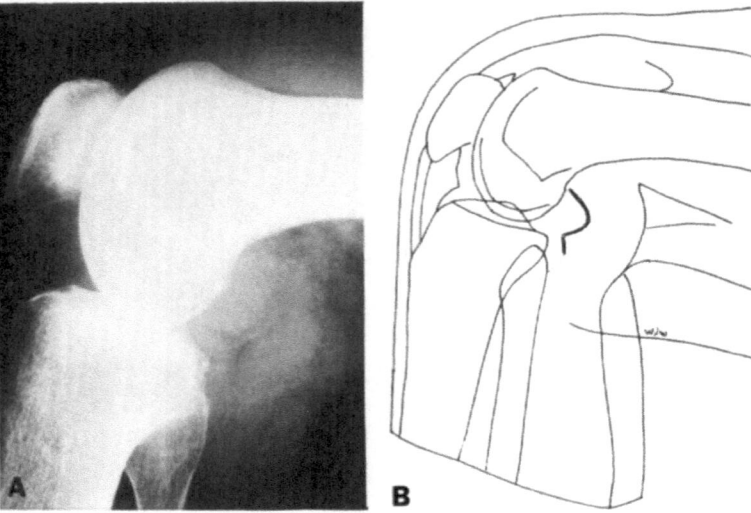

This diagnosis must always be considered when a posterior synovial component is noted in the lateral film of the knee joint.

Capsular distension may be seen in the lateral view of the knee joint in flexion in patients with rheumatoid arthritis (19). In the case shown in Figure 6-18, the capsule took on the shape of a numeral 3, which is a similar shape to that of the extrasynovial fat posteriorly.

A synovial cyst (Baker's cyst) is very common in rheumatoid disease within the popliteal fossa. Small unsuspected cysts may be demonstrated incidentally during arthrography of the knee (13). Clinically, it has been commonly observed that tense popliteal cysts are frequently associated with low pressure knee effusions, and contrast injected directly into such a cyst may not enter the cavity of the knee joint. Jayson (9) has emphasized the valvelike nature of the communication between the two cavities and the cyst has been regarded as providing a means of pressure relief for the knee (4). A popliteal cyst can be recognized as a soft tissue mass protruding posteriorly to the knee joint in the lateral view. The shadows produced by the bulky hamstrings and gastrocnemius may be confusing; but errors in diagnosis can usually be avoided by comparison with the opposite side. The posterior convexity of the mass is typical (Fig. 6-19). The cyst may extend out and be seen between the hamstrings above and the gastrocnemius below. It may come into close relationship with the deep fascia that forms the roof of the popliteal fossa. Rupture of the popliteal cyst is recognized far more commonly than rupture of any other fluid-filled synovial cavity. When this occurs, the whole calf becomes swollen, the tissue planes in the soft tissue radiograph become indistinct, and an erroneous diagnosis of deep calf vein phlebothrombosis may

Fig. 6-19. A large popliteal cyst in a young child. It protrudes posteriorly into the popliteal fossa and extends further to meet the fascia forming the roof of the fossa (arrows). The posterior convexity is typical.

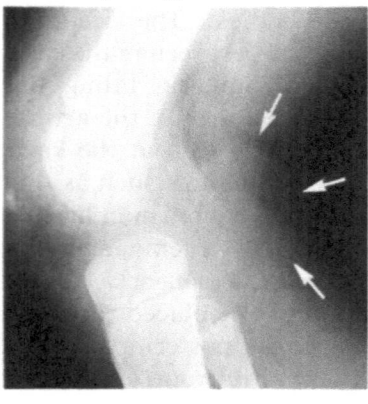

Soft Tissues of the Extremities

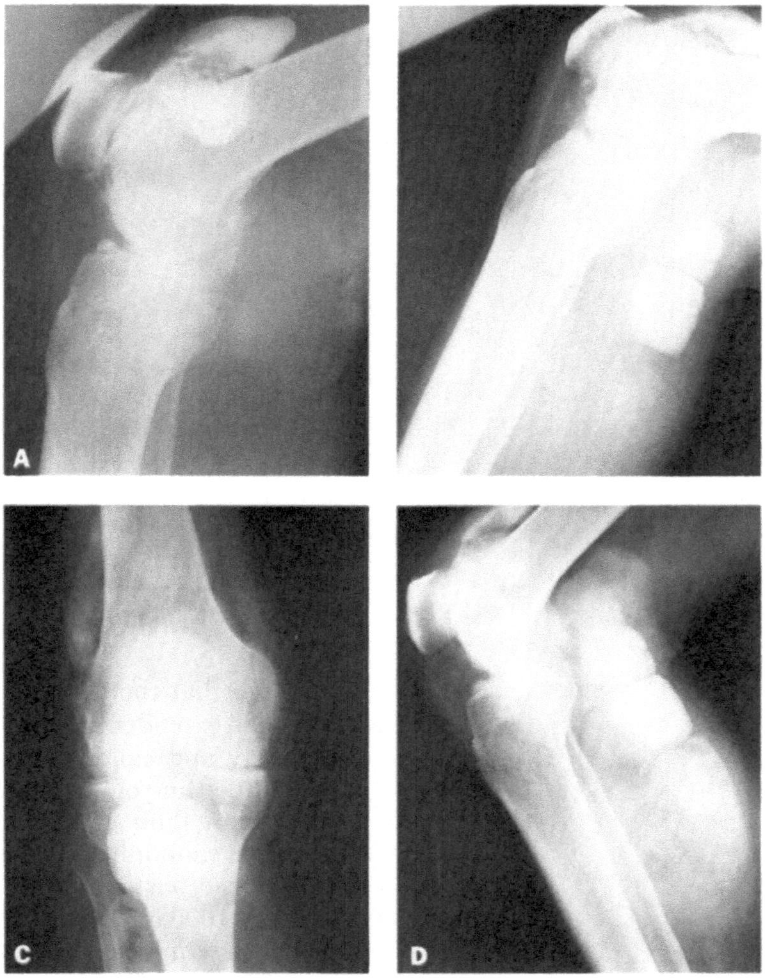

Fig. 6-20. **A.** Lateral view of an arthrogram in a rheumatoid patient showing no communication with a large popliteal cyst. The cyst appears as a soft tissue mass in the popliteal fossa. **B.** Lateral view of the same knee showing a multi-loculated popliteal cyst demonstrated by separate cyst puncture. **C.** Anteroposterior view indicating the size of the popliteal cyst and its relation to the popliteal fossa. **D.** Final lateral view when the lowest component of the cyst was separately injected.

Fig. 6-21. "Pseudorheumatoid nodule" situated in the subcutaneous tissue ventral to the infrapatellar ligament, in a 17-year-old girl without signs of a polyarthritis. Histologically such lesions are indistinguishable from a true rheumatoid nodule.

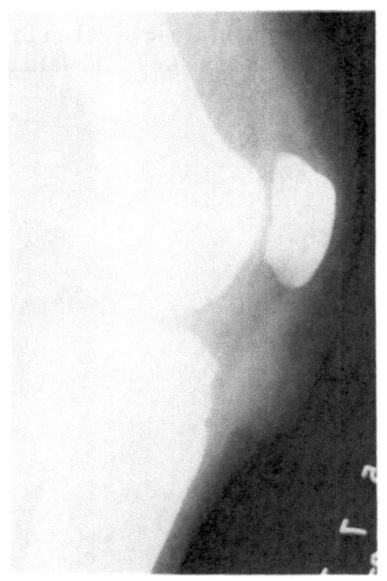

be made (8). Less commonly calf swelling, in the absence of edema, may be due to the formation of a large multiloculated cyst extending into the calf (Fig. 6-20A–D) (2,12). Free communication between the various compartments may be lost and the several components may have to be injected separately in order to demonstrate the entire structure.

Cyst formation at the rheumatoid knee, other than within the popliteal fossa, is uncommon, but anteromedial cysts are occasionally encountered which probably arise from a bursa beneath the medial ligament (14).

It is uncommon to see effusions in the prepatellar bursa in rheumatoid disease, and subcutaneous nodules at this site are also much less common than at the elbow. Nevertheless, prepatellar nodules have been recognized as the initial manifestation of rheumatoid arthritis. In children, nodules histologically similar to rheumatoid nodules, so-called pseudorheumatoid nodules, have not appeared to be the harbinger of an arthritis (Fig. 6-21) (5).

The Knee

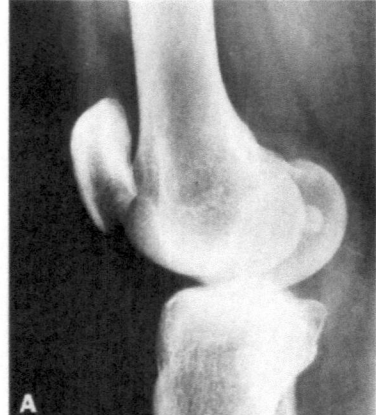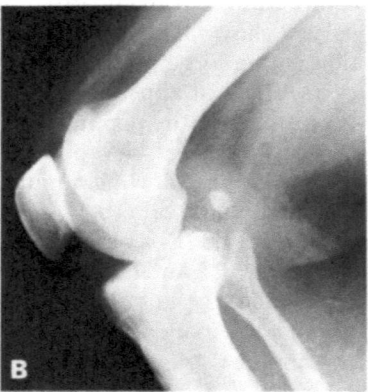

Fig. 6-22. **A.** In the extended position of the knee the fabella articulates with the femoral condyle. **B.** In the flexed position the fabella moves posteriorly and caudally.

FABELLOFEMORAL JOINT

It is noted that the fabella articulates with the femur when the knee is extended. In flexion the fabella is found to move posteriorly and caudally (Fig. 6-22A and B). If a study is made at the time of arthrography it is observed that the volume of joint fluid posteriorly increases with flexion of the joint. One cannot help feeling that the fabella and synovium are displaced posteriorly by the raised joint pressure, which may reach 1000 mm Hg. This would explain why the capsule can be seen wrapped about the fabella in some cases in flexion (Fig. 6-23A–C). Thus, it must be remembered that if the

Fig. 6-23. A normal arthrogram with three lateral views taken in extension (**A**), partial flexion (**B**), and full flexion (**C**). In the latter view the capsule is wrapped around the fabella.

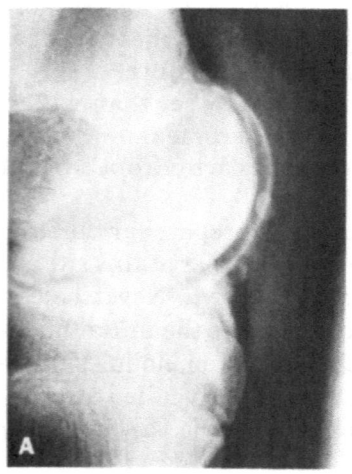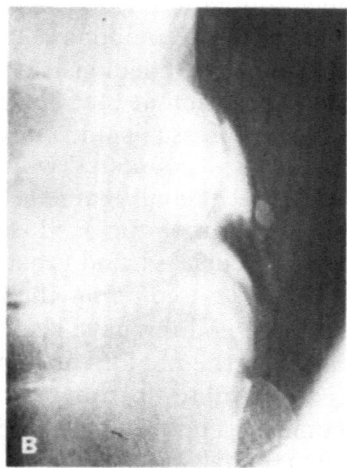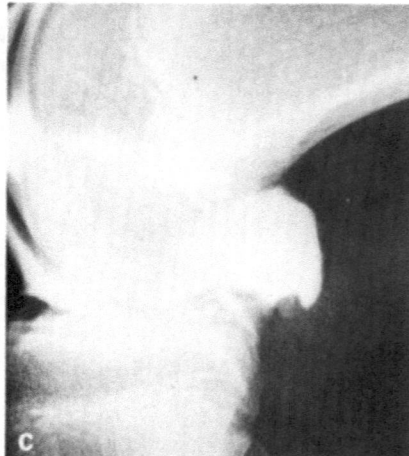

Soft Tissues of the Extremities

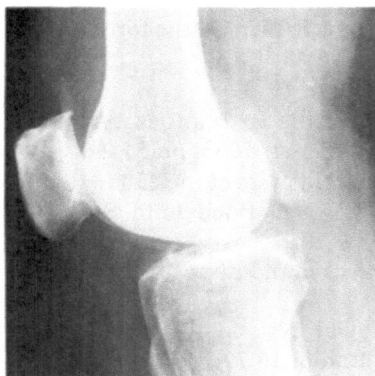

Fig. 6-24. Lipping was noted about the fabella as well as the patella, in this case of osteoarthritis. Both sesamoid bones articulate with the femur.

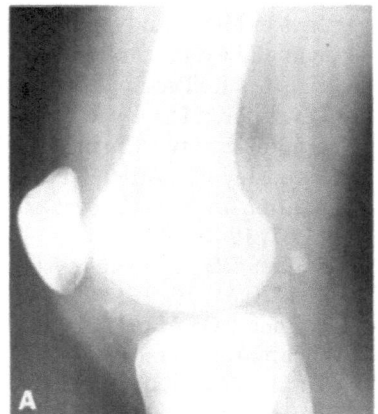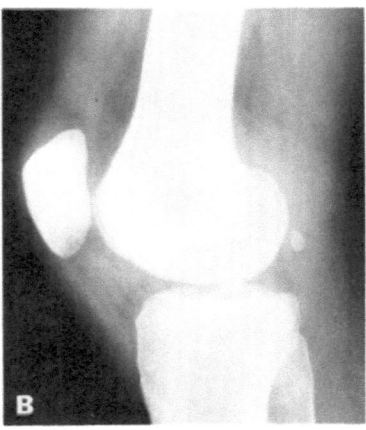

Fig. 6-25. **A.** Traumatic effusion in knee joint, with posterior capsular distension. No fracture is demonstrated. The fabella is displaced posteriorly. **B.** Knee joint on uninjured side showing the fabella in intimate relation to the femoral condyle and no joint effusion.

fabella is to be used as a marker in the lateral view, the film must be taken in almost full extension.

Lipping around the fabella may develop as part of an osteoarthritic process (Fig. 6-24).

In patients with an ossified fabella, a further sign becomes evident in a posterior effusion. The fabella is displaced posteriorly by distension of the capsule within which it lies (Fig. 6-25A and B).

References

1. Balazs EA, Watson D, Duff IF, et al: Hyaluronic acid in synovial fluid. I. Molecular parameters of hyaluronic acid in normal and arthritic human fluids. Arthritis Rheum 10:357, 1967
2. Beatty DC: Rheumatoid cysts of the calf. Proc R Soc Med 52:1106, 1959
3. Berens DL, Lin R-K: Roentgen Diagnosis of Rheumatoid Arthritis. Springfield, Ill, Thomas, 1969, pp 176–244
4. Genovese GR, Jayson MIV, Dixon AStJ: Protective value of synovial cysts in rheumatoid knees. Ann Rheum Dis 31:179, 1972
5. Greece JP, Gibson AAM: "Pseudorheumatoid" nodules in children. J Bone Joint Surg [Br] 53:724, 1971
6. Harris RD, Hecht HL: Suprapatellar effusions. A new diagnostic sign. Radiology 97:1, 1970
7. Hessen I: Fabella (sesamum genu superius laterale). Acta Radiol (Stockh) 27:177, 1946
8. Hooper JC, Brookler M: Popliteal cysts and their rupture in rheumatoid arthritis simulating thrombophlebitis. Med J Aust 1:1371, 1971

The Knee

9. Jayson MIV: Study of a valvular mechanism in the formation of synovial cysts. Ann Physiol Med 9:243, 1968
10. Kelsey CK: Personal communication, 1973
11. Lewis RW: The Knee. In Joints of the Extremities. A Radiographic Study. Springfield, Ill, Thomas, 1955, pp 56–88
12. Maudsley RH, Arden GP: Rheumatoid cysts of the calf and their relation to Baker's cyst of the knee. J Bone Joint Surg [Br] 43:87, 1961
13. Palmer DG: Synovial cysts in rheumatoid disease. Ann Intern Med 70:61, 1969
14. Palmer DG: Antero-medial synovial cysts at the knee joint in rheumatoid disease. Australas Radiol 16:79, 1972
15. Staple TW: Extrameniscal lesions demonstrated by double-contrast arthrography of the knee. Radiology 102:311, 1972
16. Taylor AR: Arthrography of the knee in rheumatoid arthritis. Br J Radiol 42:493, 1969
17. Weston WJ: Positive contrast arthrography in rheumatoid arthritis. Australas Radiol 12:141, 1968
18. Weston WJ: The extrasynovial and capsular fat pads on the posterior aspect of the knee joint. Br J Radiol 44:277, 1971
19. Weston WJ: The posterior capsule of the flexed knee joint in rheumatoid arthritis. Australas Radiol 16:89, 1972
20. Weston WJ, Anttila P: Radiographic appearance of osmium in the soft tissues of the knee in rheumatoid arthritis. Scand J Rheumatol 1:17, 1972

CHAPTER 7

The Ankle Region

RADIOLOGIC ANATOMY OF THE ANKLE JOINT

The anatomy of the synovial pouches about the ankle is the key to radiologic diagnosis in this region and must be understood before the soft tissue signs of effusions can be recognized. The synovial membrane and capsule of the ankle joint are in intimate relationship with the deep fascia and the fascia–fat interface on the medial aspect of the ankle joint. The tendon of the tibialis posterior is also closely related to the capsule here. It is in this area that the single tendon divides into its various branches. Space-occupying lesions arising from the synovial cavity are easily studied in this region because there is normally a concavity between the medial malleolus and the talus which is formed by the deep fascia, and which becomes convex when displaced. This can also be demonstrated at postmortem arthrography when the joint cavity is overdistended with a barium sulfate suspension. The distended synovial cavity, outlined by extrasynovial fat, becomes convex in outline (Fig. 7-1).

The normal synovial membrane of the ankle joint is not visible in the soft tissue radiograph. The joint space was demonstrated in 17 ankle joints by injecting barium sulfate during postmortem examination. The ankle joint is best entered with a needle directed posteriorly into one or another superior angle of the ankle mortice about 1.5 cm above and internal to the tip of the corresponding malleolus. Both an-

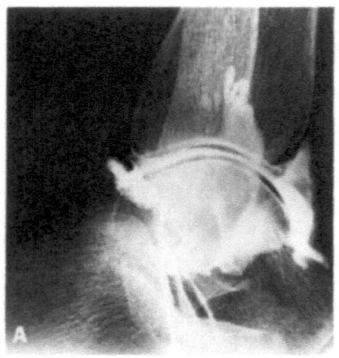

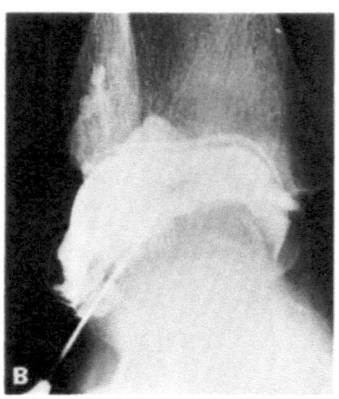

Fig. 7-1. A. Large trapezoidal type of anterior pouch of ankle joint outlined by barium at postmortem. Note extension of pouch anteriorly up onto the tibia. Lateral view.
B. Anteroposterior view of **A**.
(From Weston: Br J Radiol 31:445, 1958.)

teroposterior and lateral films were taken. Successive thin barium suspensions of 1, 3, 6, 9, and 12 ml were introduced into the joint to study the size and shape of the synovial pouches as they were distended.

The synovial cavity of the ankle extends in front of the joint, the tibia, and the talus, and varies in appearance from one person to another. Braibanti (4) and Chiappi (7) drew attention to the anterior spherical type of the distended synovial cavity, while Berridge and Bonnin (3) and Lindblom (12,13) have demonstrated a different shape, referred to here as the trapezoidal type.

The trapezoidal type is the more common (Fig. 7-1A and B). The spherical shape is seen sufficiently often, however, to be worthy of note (Fig. 7-2A and B). The trapezoidal type varies in length at its base. The reason for these two types is quite simply explained when the anteroposterior views of the arthrogram are studied. In the trapezoidal type there is a triangular extension of the synovial pouch up in front of the lower end of the tibia, which is well seen in Figure 7-1. There is a further variable extension of the pouch along the dorsal aspect of the neck of the talus. Frazer (8) drew attention to the fact that the anterior ligament of the ankle joint is very thin and consists only of a few fibers that clothe the synovial membrane. Because of this, effusions are most conspicuous anteriorly.

Posteriorly, the distended synovial pouch has a numeral 3 appearance. Braibanti (4) considered this to be due to invagination of the posterior talofibular ligament causing the synovial membrane to bulge above and below. Small prolongations of the synovial pouch are seen between the tibia and fibula which extend as far as 1.7 cm above the tibial articular surface (Figs. 7-1 and 7-2).

Fig. 7-2. A. Spherical type of anterior pouch of the ankle joint outlined by barium at postmortem. Lateral view.
B. Anteroposterior view of **A**. A small prolongation of the synovial cavity is seen extending up between the tibia and fibula.
(From Weston: Br J Radiol 31:445, 1958.)

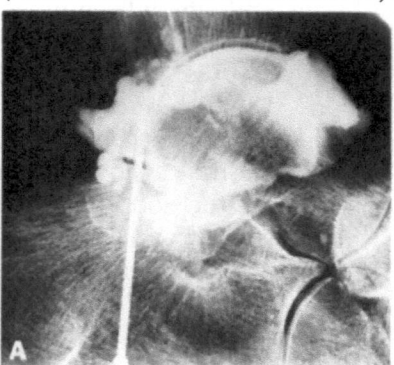

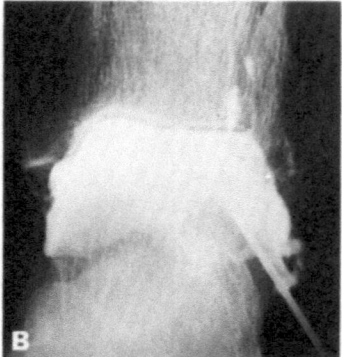

Soft Tissues of the Extremities

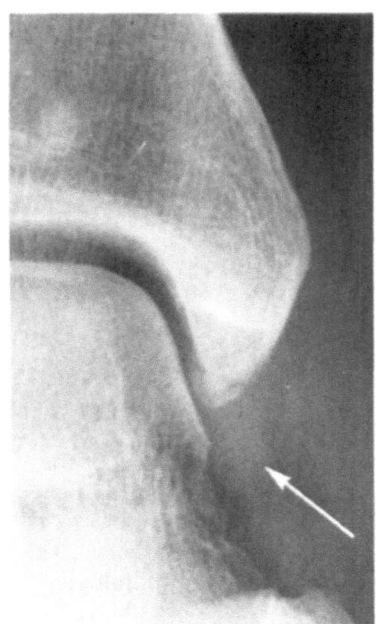

Fig. 7-3. Traumatic hemarthrosis. The space-taking synovial mass lesion is well seen in the anteroposterior view between the medial malleolus and the talus. It is convex medially (arrow). (*From Saunders and Weston: J Can Assoc Radiol 22:275, 1971.*)

In the anteroposterior view, the synovial cavity is outlined on each side of the talus. It is deeper on the lateral side, but both extensions are limited by the strong external lateral and deltoid ligaments. The upper extension between the tibia and fibula is also best seen in this view. The soft tissue signs in the lateral projection have usually been described (21) with little or no notice being taken of the synovial changes which can be seen in the anteroposterior and oblique views. Saunders and Weston (17) described the soft tissue changes in the small area between the medial malleolus and the talus which are always well seen and are worthy of particular attention.

Soft Tissue Changes

The synovial patterns that result from a variety of space-occupying lesions are similar. The changes due to distension of the ankle joint are well seen with a hemarthrosis resulting from hemophilia or trauma and with a traumatic effusion (Fig. 7-3). Weston (19) reviewed the radiographs of 605 injured ankles. Of the 304 males and the 247 females, 43.1 and 36 percent, respectively, had an effusion in the ankle joint. In 54 patients it was not possible to determine whether an effusion was present. The ratio of the trapezoidal pattern to the spherical type was 1.7:1.

Tuberculosis of the ankle joint may present with a mass lesion. The case illustrated in Figure 7-4 was associated with a small sequestrum and destructive changes were noted in the non–weight bearing portions of the joint.

An interesting case of Klippel–Trenaunay syndrome (9) was studied. A lateral soft tissue view with the leg dependent showed a large soft tissue mass on the ventral aspect of the

Fig. 7-4. A. A young Maori adult with tuberculosis of the ankle. The anterior synovial mass is well seen and the small "coke" sequestrum (arrow) is noted. Destructive changes are present in non-weight bearing areas. Lateral view. **B.** Anteroposterior view of **A.**

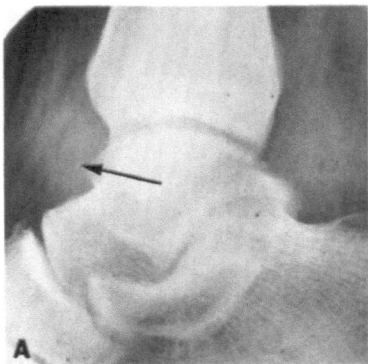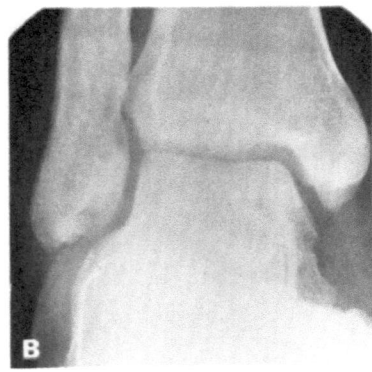

The Ankle Region

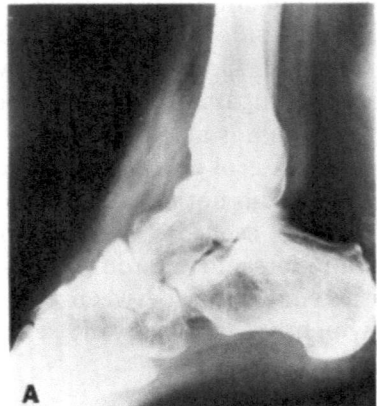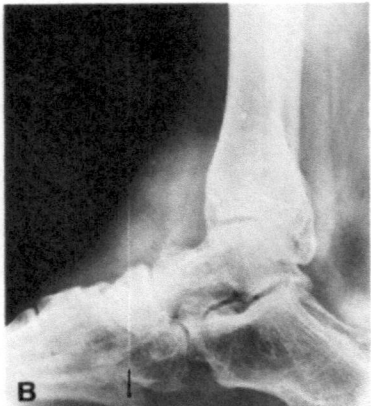

Fig. 7-5. A. Klippel–Trenaunay syndrome. Lateral view of the ankle showing a mass lesion lying anterior to ankle joint. It displaces the tendons forward. Films taken with the ankle elevated. **B.** Lateral view of the same ankle in dependency. The extrasynovial mass lesion has enlarged. This is the radiologic sign of filling.

ankle joint, deep to the deep fascia but outside the ankle joint. When the limb was elevated the soft tissue mass decreased considerably in size. This is the radiologic sign of emptying (Fig. 7-5A and B). The angiographic studies (Fig. 7-6A and B) demonstrate the vascular malformation.

A patient with a pigmented villonodular synovitis showed an unusual soft tissue pattern. A large multilobular mass

Fig. 7-6. A. Angiogram. Same case as in Figure 7-5. Arterial phase showing angiomatous malformation on the extensor aspect of ankle. **B.** Venous phase showing the enlarged venous channels of the angiomatous malformation.

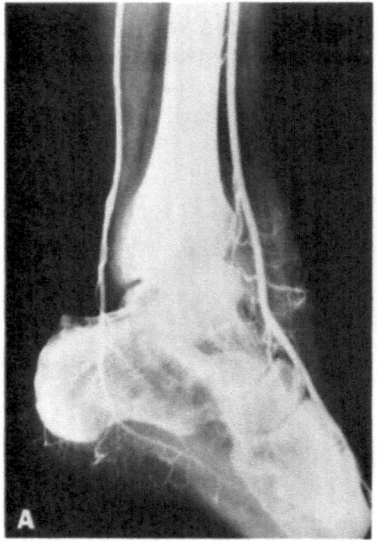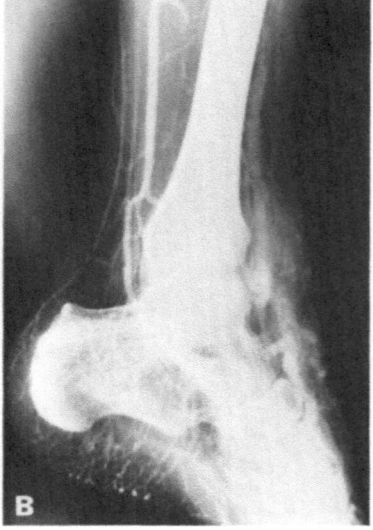

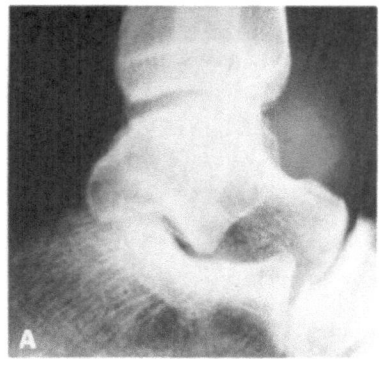

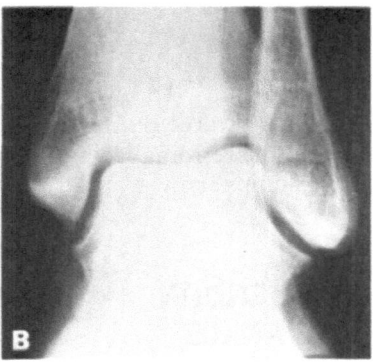

Fig. 7-7. A. Pigmented villonodular synovitis. Enlarged multilobular mass restricted to the ventral aspect of the ankle only. **B.** No evidence of a synovial mass elsewhere in the joint.

was noted on the ventral aspect of the ankle joint. There was no extension into the medial, lateral, or posterior aspects of the joint. This indicated that the synovial mass was solid and a confident diagnosis of pigmented villonodular synovitis was made. This was confirmed at surgery (Fig. 7-7A and B).

Rheumatoid Disease

Rheumatoid involvement of the ankle joint is common and the soft tissue changes follow a pattern similar to that seen with trauma, tuberculosis, septic arthritis, or hemophila—except that the synovial mass produced by rheumatoid process is often more conspicuous than in the latter conditions.

Contrast radiography of the ankle may be undertaken by introducing a 22-gauge needle into the superolateral aspect of the joint between the talus and medial aspect of the lateral malleolus. In rheumatoid disease hypertrophy of the synovium can be demonstrated and sacculation confirmed (Fig. 7-8A and B).

The soft tissue synovial mass is well seen on the plain films in both the anteroposterior and lateral views. Anteriorly, the synovial mass displaces the extensor tendons forward. Posteriorly, the mass will be seen lying deep to the flexor tendons. The latter are usually well defined posteriorly by the extrasynovial fat (Fig. 7-9).

Fig. 7-8. A. An arthrogram of the ankle joint and posterior subtalar joint involved by rheumatoid disease. The nodular hypertrophic synovium and associated sacculation has been demonstrated. Lateral view. **B.** Anteroposterior view of **A**. (*From Palmer: Ann Intern Med 70:61, 1969.*)

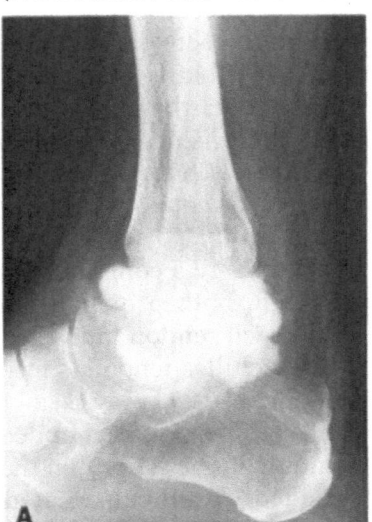
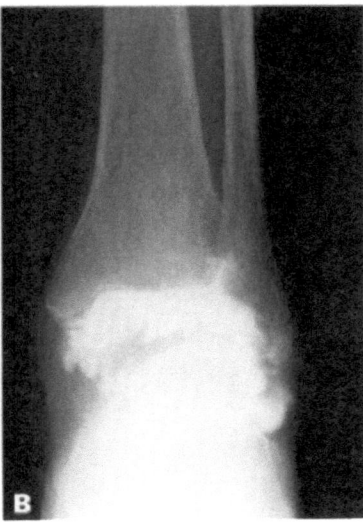

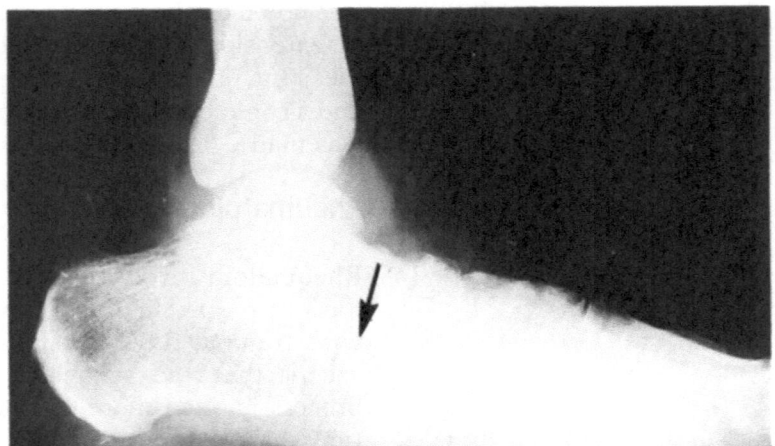

Fig. 7-9. Rheumatoid arthritis of the ankle joint. The synovial mass lesion displaces the extensor tendons forward. Posteriorly, the mass displaces the flexor tendons into the retromalleolar pad of fat. Lateral view. Note minor talar slump (arrow).

RADIOLOGIC ANATOMY OF THE TENDON SHEATHS AND BURSAE AT THE ANKLE

Fig. 7-10. Contrast injections of the tendon sheaths of tibialis anterior, extensor hallucis longus, extensor communis digitorum, and peroneus tertius. (*From Palmer: Australas Radiol 14:419, 1970.*)

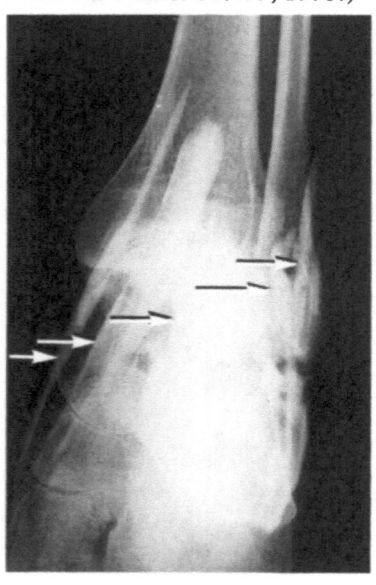

There are three groups of tendons that cross the line of the ankle joint. The associated sheaths can be demonstrated at postmortem by tenosynography, but are best defined by dissection before attempting to inject the contrast medium. The usual arrangement of these sheaths is described in the standard anatomic texts. On the anterior aspect of the ankle joint the sheath of tibialis anterior lies medially arising at a higher level than the sheath of extensor hallucis longus and the common sheath of extensor digitorum longus and peroneus tertius. The sheath of extensor hallucis longus, however, extends to the base of the first metatarsal. On the medial aspect of the ankle, the sheaths of the three tendons—tibialis posterior, flexor digitorum longus, and flexor hallucis longus—lie together with the sheath of tibialis posterior arising more proximally than the other two and that of flexor hallucis longus extending more distally, as does its extensor counterpart, as far as the base of the first metatarsal (Figs. 7-10 and 7-11). The peroneus longus and brevis tendons share a common sheath behind the lateral malleolus although, both proximally and distally, prolongations surround each tendon individually.

The Achilles tendon is inserted into the posterior aspect of the calcaneus about 2 cm from its posterosuperior angle. The tendon is not surrounded by a true sheath but, if the surrounding fascia is split on the dorsal aspect of the tendon and retracted, a well-demarcated bed is apparent. The retrocalcaneal bursa separates the Achilles tendon from the upper

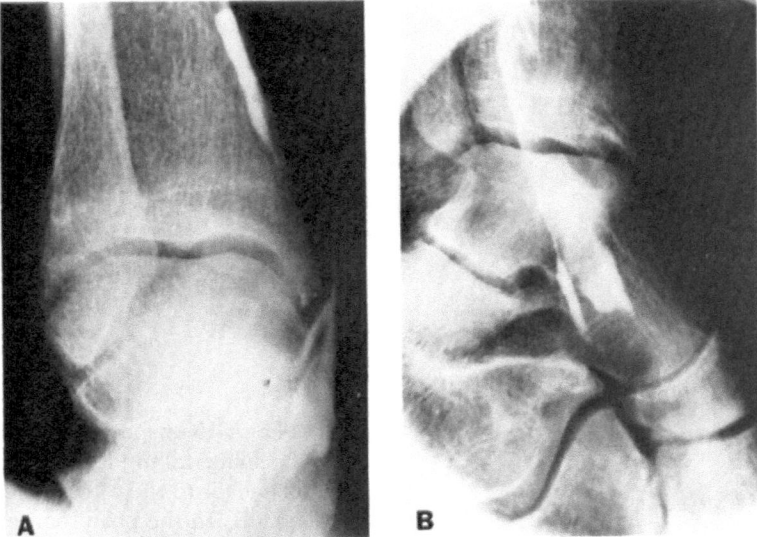

Fig. 7-11. Contrast injection of the sheath of tibialis posterior. **A.** Anteroposterior view. **B.** Oblique view.

Fig. 7-12. A normal soft tissue study of the Achilles tendon showing the extrasynovial fat of the sub-Achilles bursa. The fat is either a thin linear strip or has a triangular shape between tendon and bone (arrow). *(From Weston: Australas Radiol 14:327, 1970.)*

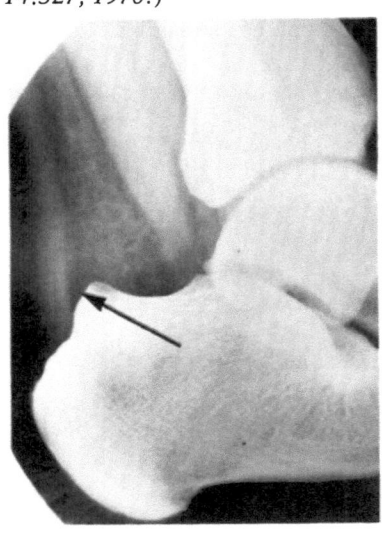

third of the dorsal surface of the calcaneus. In a normal film, the extrasynovial fat that surrounds this bursa is visible as a thin strip between the tendon and bone proximal to the insertion of the tendon (Fig. 7-12).

The anatomy of the retrocalcaneal bursa is best demonstrated by bursography. A scalp vein needle can be introduced percutaneously at postmortem examination from the posterosuperior angle of the calcaneus. The tip of the needle must remain in contact with the bone during the injection of the bursa. It can be well outlined with just 0.25 ml of barium sulfate suspension. In the lateral view, the bursa fits like a cap over the posterosuperior angle of the calcaneus. It is C-shaped, with the concavity directed forward (Fig. 7-13)(24).

Soft Tissue Changes

Nonspecific tenosynovitis involving the tendon sheaths at the ankle is less commonly recognized than at the wrist. Nevertheless, involvement of the tibialis posterior tendon (10) and peroneal tendons (20) has been recognized and calcification described (23). The soft tissue changes associated with a nonspecific peroneal tendinitis are illustrated in Figure 7-14. Nonspecific inflammatory changes with effusion into the extensor sheath are also seen. One case appeared to result from irritation of the sheath by underlying osteophytes.

Calcification of the tendons is occasionally seen (16). The

The Ankle Region

97

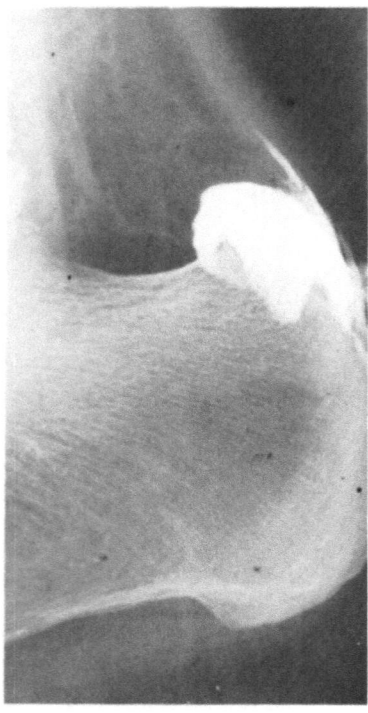

Fig. 7-13. Barium has been injected into the bursa deep to the Achilles tendon at postmortem. The bursa fits like a cap over the tuberosity of the calcaneus. Some barium has been injected into the Achilles tendon itself. (*From Weston: Australas Radiol 14:327, 1970.*)

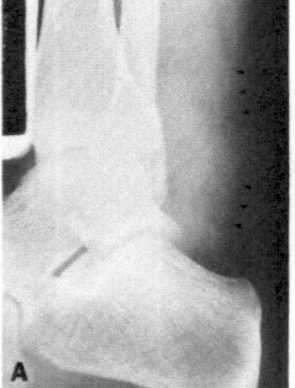 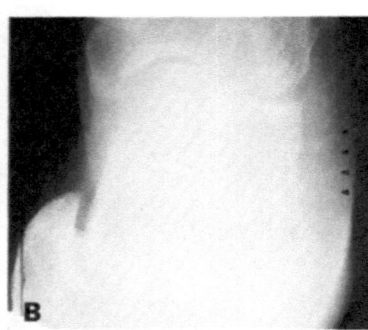

Fig. 7-14. **A.** Nonspecific peroneal tendinitis. The tendon complex acts as a space-taking lesion in the lateral view of the ankle. It extends back into the retromalleolar triangle and is wavy in outline (arrows). **B.** In the posteroanterior view of the foot, the synovial mass can be seen lateral to the calcaneus and deep to the deep fascia (arrows).

striking feature of a case of tendinitis calcarea on the dorsum of the foot was the edema that surrounded the calcification on the dorsal aspect of the tarsus (22). The initial clinical diagnosis was that of an osteomyelitis involving the tarsal bones. Four weeks later there had been considerable resorption of the calcium. The area of calcification had become smaller and denser with a well-defined border. The edema had subsided (Fig. 7-15A and B). In two further cases seen in young

Fig. 7-15. **A.** Tendinitis calcarea on the dorsum of the foot. A large ill-defined area of calcification is visible in the soft tissues on the dorsum of the left foot. There is associated soft tissue swelling. **B.** There has been considerable absorption of the calcium over a period of 4 weeks. The calcification is dense and has a well-defined border to it. The edema has subsided. (*From Weston: Br J Radiol 32:495, 1959.*)

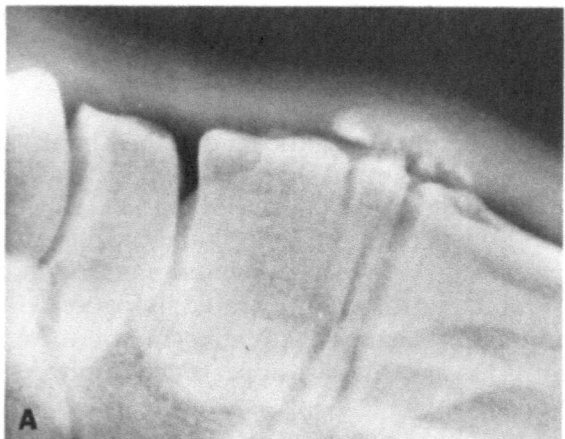 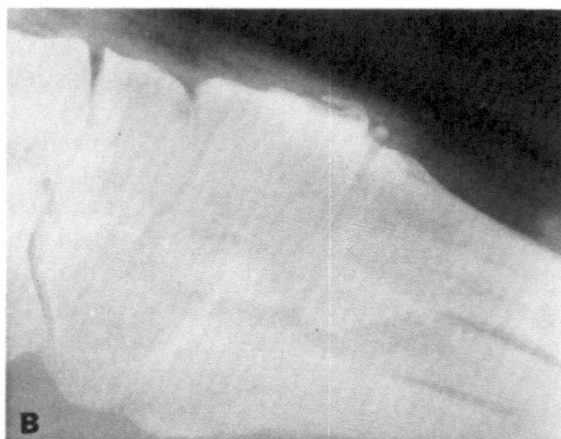

Soft Tissues of the Extremities

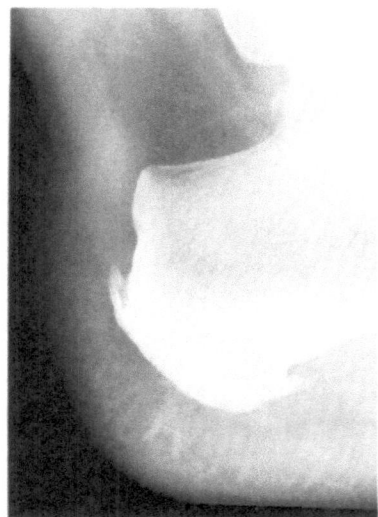

Fig. 7-16. Nonspecific thickening of the Achilles tendon just proximal to its insertion. (*From Weston: Australas Radiol 14:327, 1970.*)

Fig. 7-17. Traumatic rupture of the Achilles tendon. Marked edema is present about the tendon and in the retromalleolar triangle of fat. The ends of the tendon are visible in this example. Note air in the soft tissues, at site of incised wound.

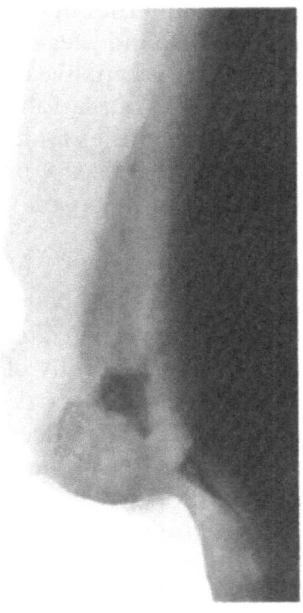

women, the areas of calcification also became smaller and the soft tissue swelling disappeared with conservative treatment.

Two cases of bilateral calcification in the tendon of peroneus longus, near the peroneal tubercle, were recorded by Lapidus (11). Miller (14) reported a case of calcareous peritendinitis of the feet in a housepainter, which he considered to be an occupational lesion related to ladder climbing. Sandstrom (16) made the following comments in his paper on peritendinitis calcarea: "In 1929, in a large amount of material from the Maria Hospital in Stockholm, I was able to demonstrate that the calcium dense shadows with which we are concerned are found not only near the shoulder joint but not infrequently in other parts of the body. The local symptoms of which the patients complain are identical wherever the localization. In my opinion we deal with a disease sui generis for which at that time I proposed the name peritendinitis calcarea."

A nonspecific tendinitis, which is often of a nodular nature, may also involve the Achilles tendon at the ankle. Such nodules involving the Achilles tendon are mainly considered to result from a partial rupture (1), but other forms of nodularity other than true rheumatoid nodules have been described, eg, pseudorheumatoid nodules in children (6) and rheumatoidlike nodules presenting as "pump bumps" (18). Occasionally, nonspecific inflammatory changes of uncertain etiology may produce considerable thickening of the tendon (Fig. 7-16).

Rupture of the Achilles tendon can occur as a spontaneous rupture or can follow direct trauma. The clear outline of the tendon is lost and edema can be seen in the retromalleolar triangle and in the overlying subcutaneous tissues. The normally taut tendon becomes slack and develops a concavity toward the tibia. It is usually difficult to identify the ends of the tendons because of the edema (Fig. 7-17). A good description of this lesion can be found in an article by Revend and Kittleson (15).

Rheumatoid Disease

Bywaters (5) described the associated soft tissue changes about the heel. He stated that "the earliest radiological sign of a sub-Achilles lesion is in the soft tissues. The tendon becomes thicker in the lateral view and the clear space beneath it, normally occupied by radiolucent fat, becomes opaque owing to the presence of inflammatory cells, fluid, and blood vessels." Vainio (19) noted that the first radiographic sign of an Achilles bursitis is a swelling of the soft tissue producing an appearance "as if the Achilles tendon has been pushed away from the bone." Berens and Lin (2) stated that "the earliest soft tissue finding is an area of edema of water density

The Ankle Region

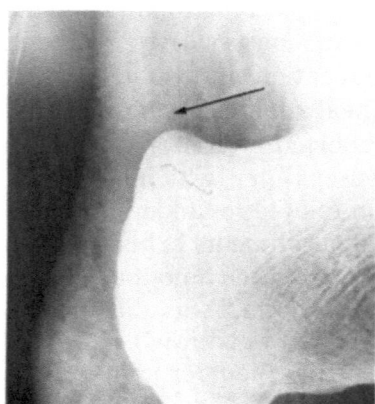

Fig. 7-18. The enlarged sub-Achilles bursa is displacing the Achilles tendon posteriorly (arrow). The extrasynovial fat around the bursa can still be defined. This patient had recently developed rheumatoid arthritis. *(From Weston: Australas Radiol 14:327, 1970.)*

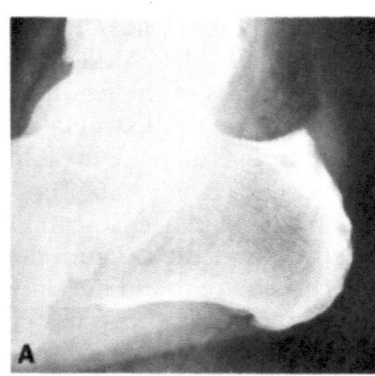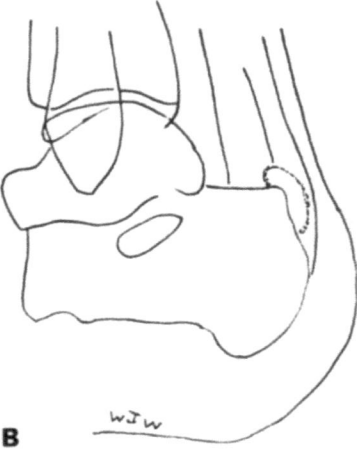

Fig. 7-19. A. An enlarged right sub-Achilles bursa with clearly defined extrasynovial fatty layer, in a patient with rheumatoid arthritis. An erosion is noted in the underlying bone. Edema is present in the retromalleolar triangle of fat. **B.** Line diagram of **A.** *(From Weston: Australas Radiol 14:327, 1970.)*

Fig. 7-20. Multiple nodules in Achilles tendon, just distal to the muscle bellies. The tendon is also thickened just proximal to its insertion.

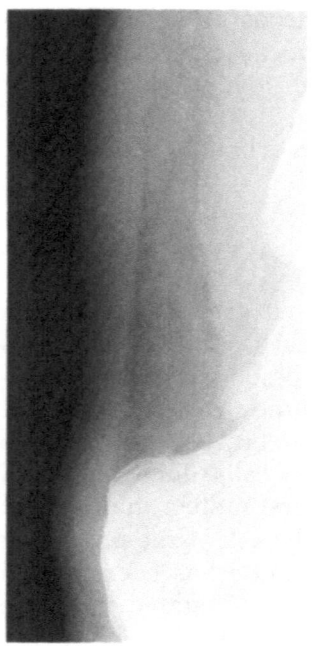

encroaching upon the pre-Achilles tendon fat pad at the superior surface of the os calcis."

When the retrocalcaneal bursa is involved by rheumatoid disease, a rounded mass is seen to fill the angle between the Achilles tendon and the upper margin of the tuberosity of the calcaneus. The extrasynovial fat surrounding the bursa is displaced by the synovial fluid, fibrin bodies, synovial hypertrophy, and edema. In the early case, the extrasynovial fat about this enlarged bursa will be seen on a fine grained film (Fig. 7-18). The cephalic margin of the enlarged bursa, seen in the angle between the Achilles tendon and the superior surface of the calcaneus, is smooth and convex and is easily identified in the lateral view. The preerosive and erosive changes in the cortex of the calcaneus deep to the bursa follow the early soft tissue changes (Fig. 7-19). The Achilles tendon can itself become thickened at a later stage in the disease process. Subcutaneous rheumatoid nodules may form on the dorsal surface of the tendon (Fig. 7-20).

Distension of the peroneal and flexor sheaths by effusion fluid produces characteristic arcuate swellings behind the malleoli. A distended extensor sheath is constricted centrally by the inferior retinaculum. Tenosynography of these sheaths, when distended by fluid, is a straightforward procedure. The sheath may be entered with a 22-gauge needle, introduced at an acute angle to the skin in the line of the sheath. Some (1 to 3 ml) fluid can usually be withdrawn and replaced by a similar quantity of 60 percent urografin which will produce good contrast. The nodularity of the hypertrophied rheumatoid synovium already noted in the tendon sheaths in-

Soft Tissues of the Extremities

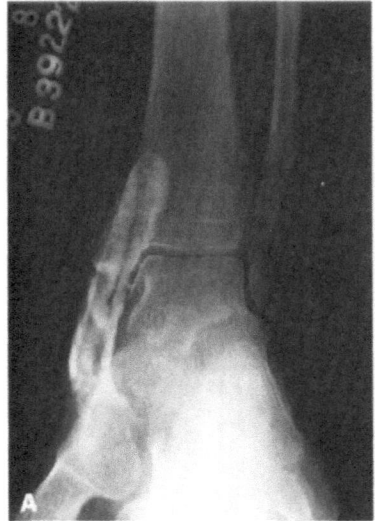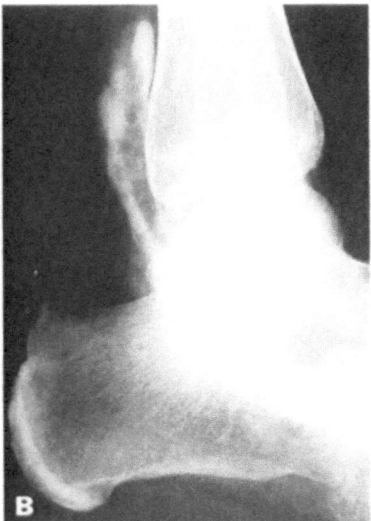

Fig. 7-21. A. The sheath of tibialis posterior involved by rheumatoid arthritis, outlined with 60 percent urografin. Anteroposterior view. **B.** Lateral view of **A.** *(From Palmer: Australas Radiol 14:419, 1970.)*

volved by rheumatoid at the wrist will again be seen (Figs. 7-21 and 7-22).

RADIOLOGIC ANATOMY OF THE SOFT TISSUES OF THE HEEL PAD

The heel pad is the best anatomic site to study the cutis line and the fascia–fat interface. Running from the deep fascia to the cutis line are vertical strands of connective tissues which carry the neurovascular pedicles of the skin. Some of these columns are linked by horizontal bands of fibrous connective tissue.

By study of the angiographic features of the heel one can understand this pattern of connective tissue columns. In Figure 7-23 the numerous arterial and venous trunks can be seen running to and from the cutis line in the sole of the foot. Chambers of fat lie between these fibrous connective tissue columns. These chambers of fat distribute the body weight transmitted through the lower limbs. It is these columns of fat that cushion the stresses applied to the feet with walking, running, and other athletic exercises.

Soft Tissue Changes

In an osteomyelitis of the calcaneus swelling of these connective tissue columns that run from the cutis line to the deep fascia of the foot will be seen together with some increase in

The Ankle Region

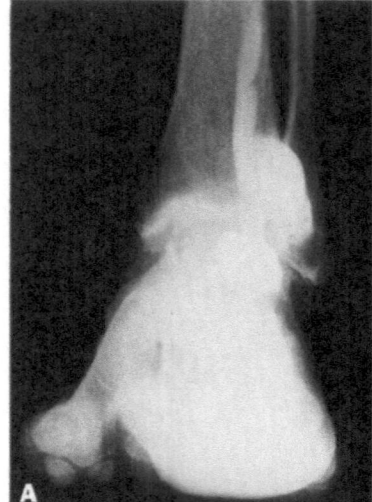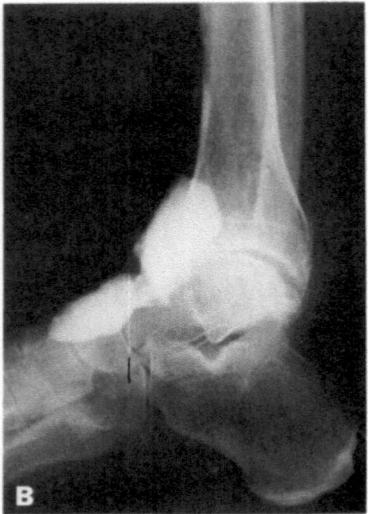

Fig. 7-22. A. A fluctuant swelling on the extensor aspect of the ankle shown by contrast examination to be due to sacculation from the sheath of extensor hallucis longus. The patient had rheumatoid arthritis. Anteroposterior view. **B.** Lateral view of **A**. (*From Palmer: Australas Radiol 14:419, 1970.*)

Fig. 7-23. An angiogram showing the arterial and venous trunks running from the deep fascia to the cutis line in the sole of the foot. These vascular channels lie in the fibrous connective tissue columns connecting the deep fascia to the epithelium.

Fig. 7-24. Patient with rheumatoid nodule in heel pad. The nodule is roughly circular and is homogeneous in texture (arrow). The thickness of the heel pad is increased. Synovial reaction noted in ankle joint.

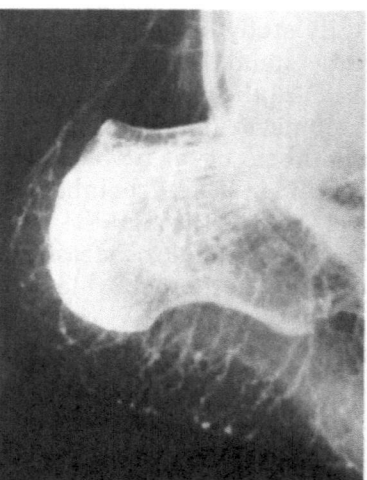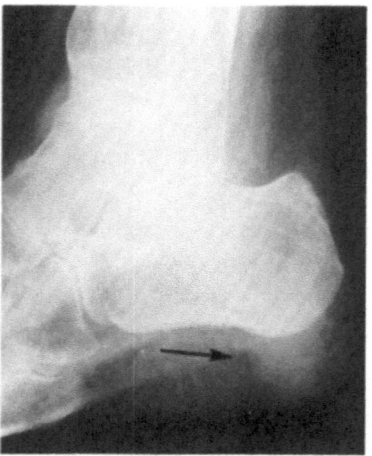

the thickness of the heel pad. This combined pattern is an important early radiologic sign of osteomyelitis of the calcaneus. Edema of the retromalleolar triangle is usually associated.

Rheumatoid Disease

Rheumatoid nodules may develop in the heel pads (Fig. 7-24). These nodules can be bilateral. Such nodules act as space-taking lesions that surround and obliterate the fibrous connective tissue columns that run from the deep fascia to the cutis line. They form a dense homogeneous mass which contrasts with the pattern of the connective tissue columns, and are roughly circular in outline. Associated erosion of the inferior surface of the calcaneus may be present. The thickness of the heel pad is increased. Obesity alone will increase this thickness but does not change the pattern of fibrous columns seen in this area. The changes of acromegaly can be similar.

References

1. Auquier L, Siaud JR: Tendinitis nodulaires du tendon d'Achille. Rev Rhum 38:373, 1971
2. Berens DL, Lin R-K: Roentgen Diagnosis of Rheumatoid Arthritis. Springfield, Ill, Thomas, 1969, pp 137–159
3. Berridge FR, Bonnin JG: The radiographic examination of the ankle joint including arthrography. Surg Gynecol Obstet 79:383, 1944
4. Braibanti T: Contribute all conoscenza dell' aspetto radiologico della parti molli. Ann Radiol Diagn 19:102, 1947
5. Bywaters EGL: Heel lesions of rheumatoid arthritis. Ann Rheum Dis 13:42, 1954
6. Caughey DE, Calabro JJ, Gracchiolo A: Benign rheumatoid (pseudorheumatoid) nodules in children. Arthritis Rheum 12:285, 1969
7. Chiappi S: Studio radiologica sulle parti molli articolori e periarticolari. Le parti molli dell' articolazione tibiotarsua nel quandro normali e nelli lesioni da trauma. Radiol Med 38:621, 1952
8. Frazer JE: The Joints of the Foot In Buchanan's Manual of Anatomy, 6th ed. London, Balliere, 1937, p 665
9. Klippel M, Trenaunay P: Du naevus variqueux osteohypertrophique. Arch Gen Med 77:641, 1900
10. Langenskiold A: Chronic nonspecific tenosynovitis of the tibialis posterior tendon. Acta Orthop Scand 38:301, 1967
11. Lapidus PW: Infiltration therapy of acute tendinitis with calcification. Surg Gynecol Obstet 76:715, 1943
12. Lindblom K: Arthrography. J Faculty Radiol 3:151, 1952

13. Lindblom K: Arthrography. In McLaren JW (ed) Modern Trends in Diagnostic Radiology, 2nd Series. London, Butterworth, 1953, pp 251–266

14. Miller CF: Occupational calcaneous peritendinitis of the feet. Am J Roentgenol 61:506, 1949

15. Revend PM, Kittleson AC: Spontaneous Achilles tendon rupture. Radiology 93:1341, 1969

16. Sandstroem C: Peritendinitis calcarea, A common disease of middle life. Its diagnosis, pathology, and treatment. Am J Roentgenol 40:1, 1938

17. Saunders CG, Weston WJ: Synovial mass lesions in anteroposterior projection of the ankle joint. J Can Assoc Radiol 22:275, 1971

18. Sturgill BC, Allan JH: Rheumatoid-like nodules presenting as "Pump Bumps" in a patient without rheumatoid arthritis. Arthritis Rheum 13:175, 1970

19. Vainio K: The rheumatoid foot. A clinical study with pathological and roentgenological comments. Ann Chir Gynaecal Fenn (Suppl) 1:16, 1956

20. Webster FS: Peroneal tenosynovitis with pseudo tumour. J Bone Joint Surg [Am] 50:143, 1968

21. Weston WJ: Traumatic effusions of the ankle joint and posterior subtaloid joints. Br J Radiol 31:445, 1958

22. Weston WJ: Tendinitis calcarea on the dorsum of the foot. Br J Radiol 32:495, 1959

23. Weston WJ: Peroneal tendinitis calcarea. Br J Radiol 32:134, 1959

24. Weston WJ: The bursa deep to tendo Achilles. Australas Radiol 14:327, 1970

Soft Tissues of the Extremities

CHAPTER 8

The Tarsus and Foot

RADIOLOGIC ANATOMY OF THE POSTERIOR SUBTALAR JOINT

The synovial pouch of the posterior subtalar joint is again best studied in the lateral view. The joint cavity starts behind the sinus tarsi and runs posteriorly out along the upper surface of the calcaneus, extending on to both its lateral and medial aspects. It is significant that during arthrography this joint is sometimes outlined at the same time as the ankle joint. Hansson (2) noted that there was communication between the ankle joint and subtalar joint in 4 out of his 48 cases studied by arthrography. This communication was often found during postmortem arthrography when the ankle joint was fully distended (Fig. 8-1A and B) (5). The joint space variable is but in all cases extends posterior to that of the ankle joint, sometimes almost reaching the Achilles tendon.

Soft Tissue Changes

Trauma at the ankle may be associated with effusion into the posterior subtalar joint. This was seen in 36 of 605 such patients (6 percent) (Fig. 8-2) (5). It is important to recognize that there is a plane of fat between the synovial mass and the tuberosity of the calcaneus. This is the extrasynovial fat which separates the sausage-shaped synovial pouch from the

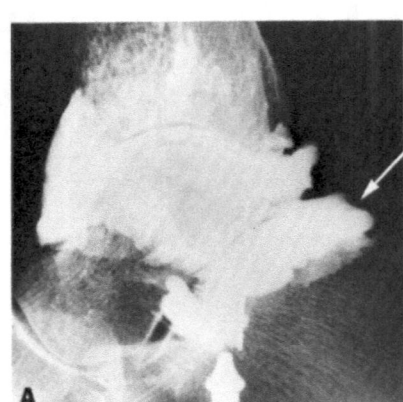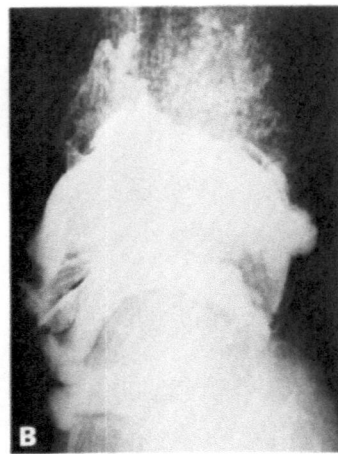

Fig. 8-1. A. Lateral view of a large trapezoidal type of anterior pouch of the ankle joint outlined by barium at postmortem. The posterior compartment of the subtaloid joint has been outlined as well (arrow). In the latter the synovial cavity extends back along the tuberosity of the calcaneus. Some barium has entered the veins in the tibia and soft tissues. **B.** Anteroposterior view of **A**. (*From Weston: Br J Radiol 31:445, 1958.*)

upper surface of the tuberosity of the calcaneus. It forms a space-filling lesion in the caudal region of the triangular retromalleolar fat pad.

Rheumatoid Disease

In patients with rheumatoid involvement of the posterior subtalar joint a synovial mass lesion is noted in the posterior malleolar triangle which is in intimate relationship with the tuberosity. The pattern is similar to that seen in trauma, but the soft tissue mass is usually larger than that seen in trau-

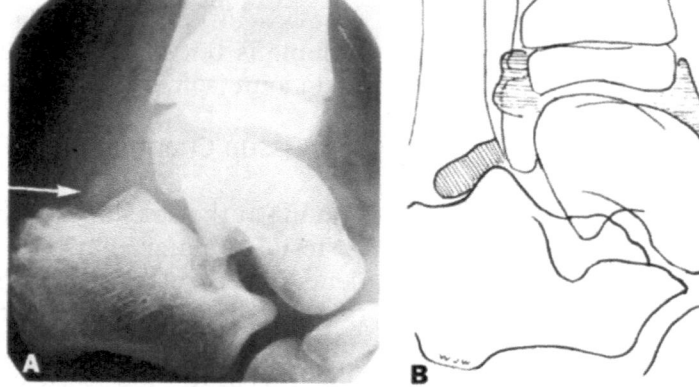

Fig. 8-2. A. There is a moderate sized trapezoidal type of traumatic effusion in the ankle joint. There is associated effusion into the posterior subtaloid joint (arrow) and edema in the retromalleolar triangle. **B.** Line drawing of **A**. (*From Weston: Br J Radiol 31:445, 1958.*)

Soft Tissues of the Extremities

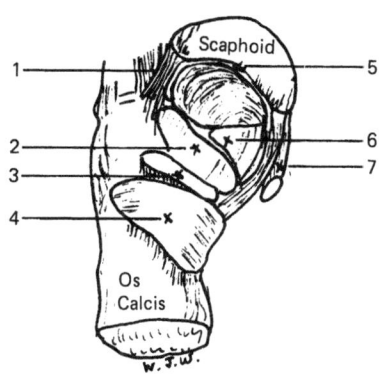

Fig. 8-3. Line drawing of the articular cup for the head of the talus of the anterior talocalcaneonavicular joint. 1, calcaneonavicular part of the Y-shaped ligament of Chopart; 2, calcaneal facet for the anterior talocalcaneonavicular joint; 3, interosseous ligament; 4, posterior facet for talocalcaneal joint; 5, insertion of dorsal talonavicular ligament; 6, plantar calcaneonavicular ligament; 7, tendon of tibialis posterior. *(From Weston: Australas Radiol 13:365, 1969.)*

matic cases. An effusion due to rheumatoid arthritis in this joint has been demonstrated by Lewis (3).

THE RADIOLOGIC ANATOMY OF THE TALOCALCANEONAVICULAR JOINT

The talocalcaneonavicular joint is the largest and most important diathrodial joint in the tarsus. The head of the talus articulates with the navicular, the anterior surface of the calcaneus, and the dorsal surface of the calcaneonavicular ligament (spring ligament). This ligament extends upward on the medial aspect of the joint. Laterally, the outer wall of the articular cup for the head of the talus is completed by the calcaneonavicular portion of the Y-shaped ligament of Chopart (Fig. 8-3).

The articular capsule is thickened posteriorly to form the interosseous ligament in the sinus tarsi between the talus and the calcaneus. The dorsal talonavicular ligament connects the neck of the talus to the dorsal surface of the navicular. According to Beetham et al (1) "The articular capsule and the synovial membrane of the anterior talocalcaneonavicular joint are tightly bound to the bones composing the joint; and allow little, if any, distension of the articular cavity." However, this joint will hold 4 to 5 ml of contrast medium, indicating that the joint cavity is moderately large and can be distended. This agrees with the anatomic description that the joint capsule is imperfectly developed.

This joint is best injected from the medial aspect of the foot just proximal to the tuberosity of the navicular. The interval between the tendons of tibialis posterior and tibialis anterior is the guide to the optimal site for puncture of the joint. The articular surface of the navicular can be palpated between these two tendons.

The synovial cavity demonstrated by the arthrogram extends up to the level of the dorsal aspect of the neck of the talus. A thin layer of opaque medium is also seen between the head of the talus and the navicular (Fig. 8-4A and B) (9).

Soft Tissue Changes

An effusion or hemarthrosis produces a soft tissue synovial mass on the dorsal aspect of the talonavicular joint which is seen in the lateral view. Such a soft tissue mass is sometimes seen on the dorsal aspect of the talonavicular joint after injury to the ankle region. This mass displaces the extensor tendons toward the dorsum of the joint. As the effusion or hemarthrosis is absorbed the soft tissue mass becomes smaller.

The Tarsus and Foot

107

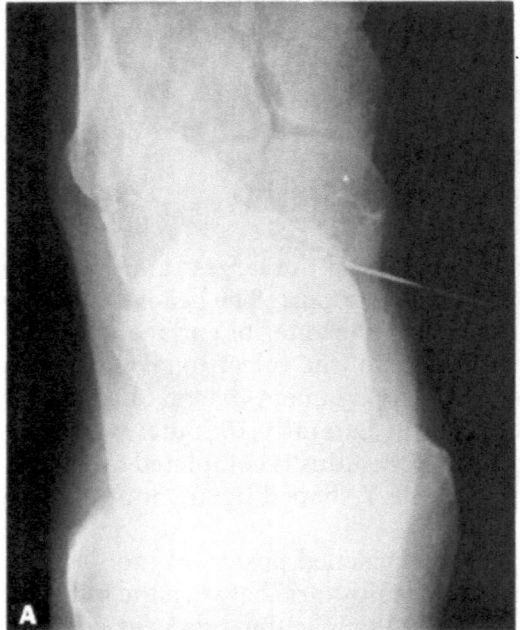 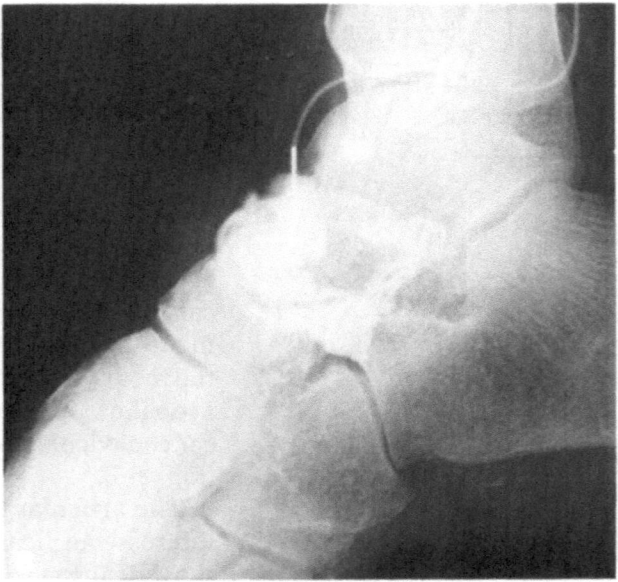

Fig. 8-4. **A.** Posteroanterior view of an arthrogram of the anterior talocalcaneonavicular joint. The contrast medium in the articular cup for the head of the talus is well shown. **B.** Lateral view of **A**. (*From Weston: Australas Radiol 13:365, 1969.*)

Rheumatoid Disease

When the talocalcaneonavicular joint is involved in rheumatoid disease a soft tissue mass may be seen on the radiograph in the lateral view of the foot, which is best assessed while bearing weight (12). Such a synovial mass lesion causes displacement of the extrasynovial fat pads from their normal position over the head and neck of the talus toward the dorsum of the foot. The extensor tendons and their sheaths are in turn displaced (Fig. 8-5).

The synovial changes vary in degree. In Still's disease the changes are often striking, for the midtarsal synovial mass may meet that from the ankle joint. Under these circumstances the synovial masses are separated by two layers of extrasynovial fat, ie, one about the ankle joint synovium and the other about the talonavicular synovium (Fig. 8-6).

These synovial changes may of course be associated with osteoporosis, erosion, cartilage loss, and subluxation of the joint. Both the posteroanterior and oblique views of the foot together with the lateral weight-bearing view are helpful in assessing the bony and cartilaginous changes. Vainio (4a) noted that the midtarsal joint was involved in 66 percent of cases of rheumatoid disease. The head of the talus becomes subluxed in the plantar direction in some patients, with

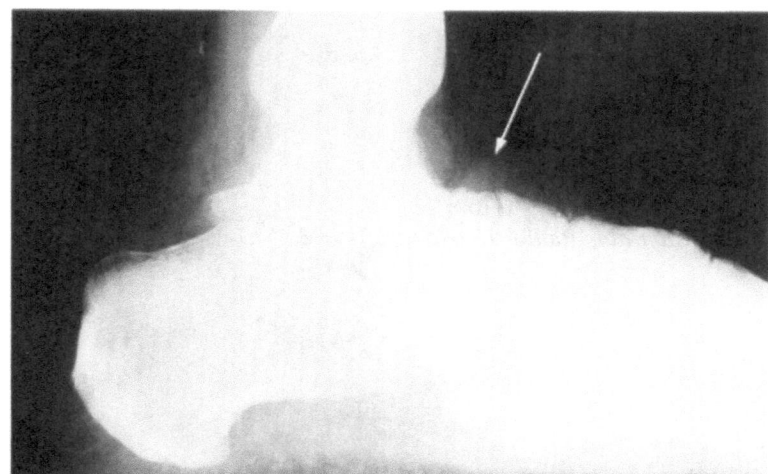

Fig. 8-5. The synovial mass lesion in the lateral view of the talocalcaneonavicular joint is seen on the dorsal aspect of the head and neck of the talus (arrow). This mass is outlined dorsally by extrasynovial fat. It displaces the extensor tendons away from the midtarsal joint.

development of a flat foot (talar slump) (Fig. 8-7). This is similar to the change seen in the carpus in rheumatoid arthritis when there is an ulnar drift of the seaphoid.

Fig. 8-6. A large synovial mass lesion in the ankle joint and anterior talocalcaneonavicular joint. The individual synovial masses are in contact on the dorsal aspect of the head and neck of the talus. They are separated by two layers of extrasynovial fat. This patient had juvenile rheumatoid arthritis. (*From Weston: Australas Radiol 16:84, 1972.*)

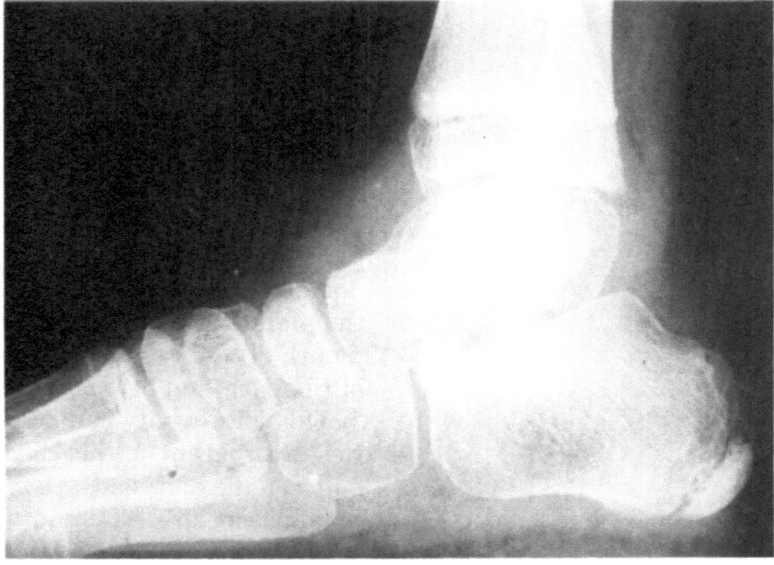

Fig. 8-7. A. The head of the talus is subluxed (arrow) in a plantar direction in the erect lateral weight-bearing view. This is the talar slump and leads to a flat foot. **B.** Line drawing of **A**. (*From Weston: Australas Radiol 16:84, 1972.*)

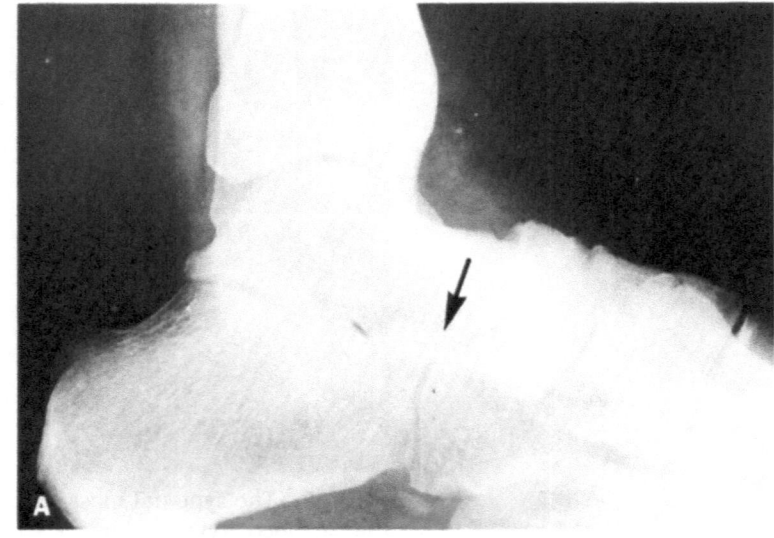

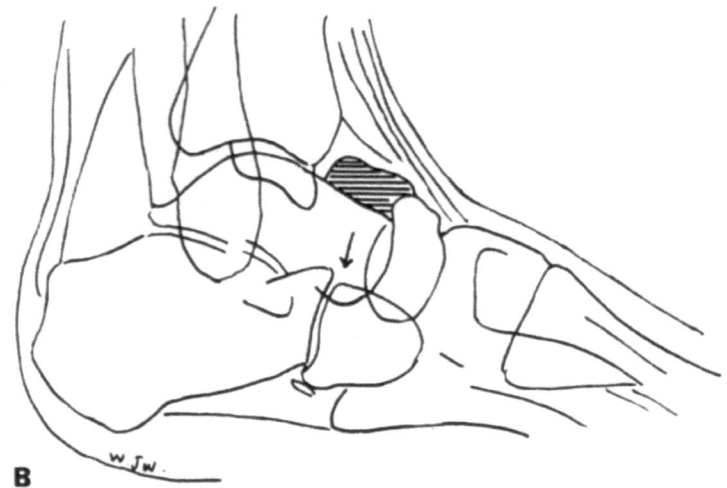

RADIOLOGIC ANATOMY OF THE CALCANEOCUBOID JOINT

The calcaneocuboid joint is a saddle-shaped diarthrodial joint with a capsule that is imperfectly developed. There are four strengthening ligaments which are as follows: (1) the dorsal calcaneocuboid ligament (a thin broad ligament); (2) the plantar calcaneocuboid ligament (the short plantar ligament); (3) the calcaneocuboid part of the Y-shaped ligament of Chopart; and (4) the long plantar ligament.

This joint cavity can hold 1.5 ml of opaque medium. On the arthrogram a thin layer of contrast medium is seen between the bone ends. Recesses are noted on the dorsal and plantar aspects of the joint (Fig. 8-8A and B).

This joint is best approached from the lateral aspect of the

Fig. 8-8. A. Posteroanterior view of an arthrogram of the calcaneocuboid joint. The saddle-shaped facets and the dorsal and plantar recesses are noteworthy features of this joint. **B.** Lateral view of **A**. (*From Weston: Australas Radiol 16:84, 1972.*)

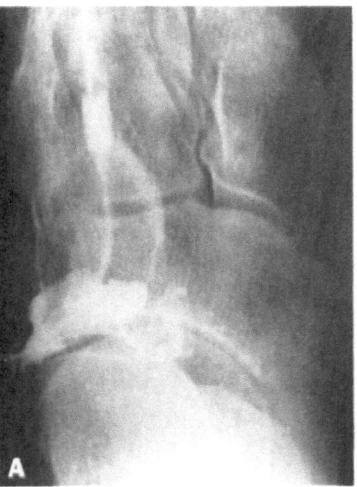
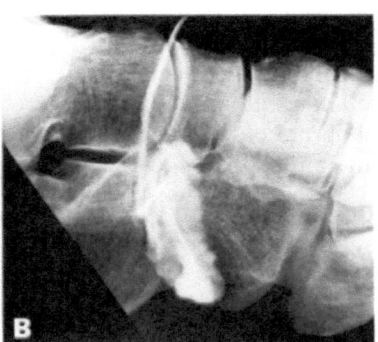

foot. The peroneal tendons about the peroneal tubercle are landmarks. The needle is inserted into the joint, which can be palpated distal and dorsal to the peroneal tubercle and the tendons. The level of the joint laterally corresponds to that of the tuberosity of the navicular medially. The calcaneal margin of the joint can be palpated in the gap between the extensor tendons dorsomedially and the peroneal tendons inferolaterally (9).

Soft Tissue Changes

Perhaps surprisingly a synovial effusion as a result of trauma has not been noted in this joint.

Rheumatoid Disease

In rheumatoid arthritis one may see a synovial mass on the lateral aspect of the calcaneocuboid joint. This mass is usually quite small because of the robust articular ligaments.

RADIOLOGIC ANATOMY OF THE METATARSOPHALANGEAL AND INTERPHALANGEAL JOINTS OF THE TOES

The anatomy and the arthrographic appearances of the metatarsophalangeal and interphalangeal joints are similar to those of the comparable finger joints (Figs. 8-9A–C, 8-10A and B, 8-11A and B) (8). The normal metatarsophalangeal joint has a capsule that is closely applied to the base of the proximal phalanx and to the head of the metatarsal. The joint capsule is shaped like a box (Fig. 8-9D).

Fig. 8-9. **A.** Postmortem arthrogram of second metatarsophalangeal joint. **B.** PM arthrogram of fifth metatarsophalangeal joint. **C.** PM arthrogram of the second and first metatarsophalangeal joints. **D.** Line diagram of the second metatarsophalangeal joint. The joint capsule is shaped like a box. (*From Weston: Australas Radiol 13:211, 1969.*)

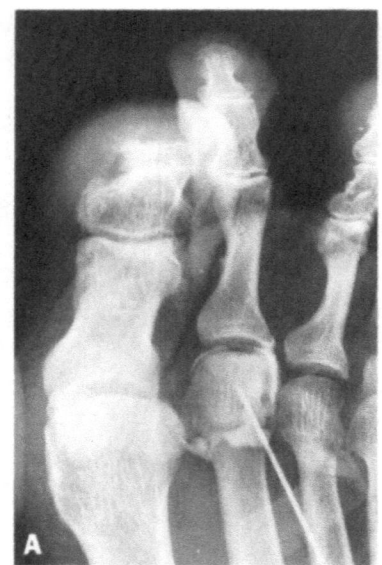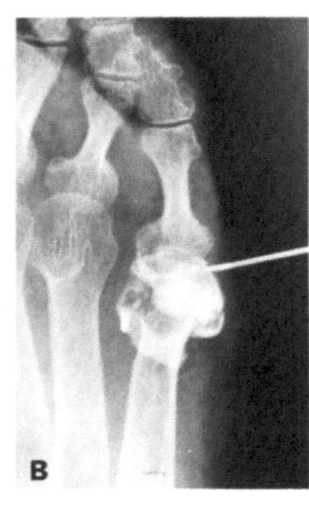

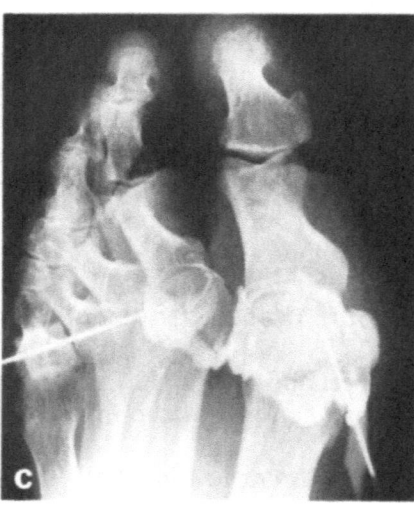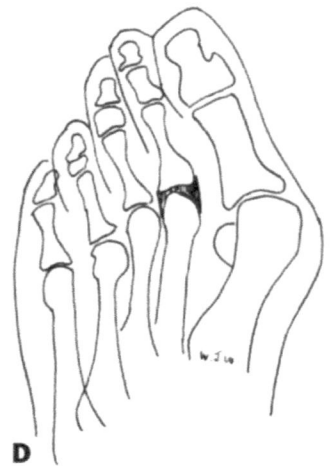

Fig. 8-10. **A.** Posteroanterior projection of the arthrogram of the proximal interphalangeal joint of the second toe, at postmortem. **B.** Oblique projection of **A**. (*From Weston: Australas Radiol 13:211, 1969.*)

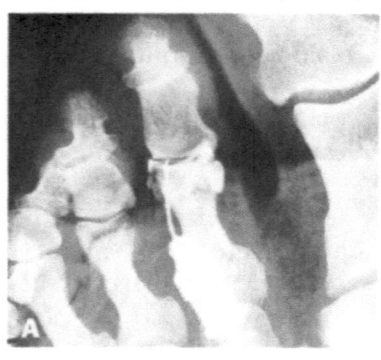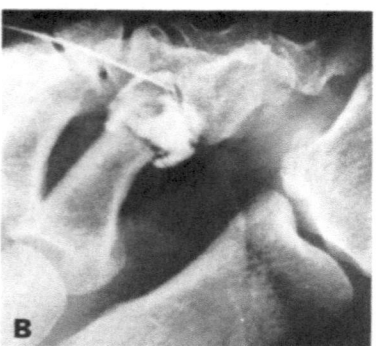

Soft Tissue Changes

Joint space widening can often be recognized when intracapsular fractures involve the metatarsophalangeal and interphalangeal joints of the toes of children; but it is not usually seen in adults. It is postulated that this joint space widening results from a hemarthrosis (10). For this to occur the synovial membrane and probably the capsule as well must be intact. The periosteum may be elevated as a result of the intracapsular fracture reaching the periosteum. The periosteum is much thicker in children than in adults and thus is less likely to tear. After 2 to 4 weeks the joint width returns to normal and early callus formation will be seen at the fracture site (Fig. 8-12).

Soft Tissues of the Extremities

Fig. 8-11. **A.** Posteroanterior projection of the normal arthrogram of the interphalangeal joint of the great toe at postmortem. **B.** Lateral projection of **A**. (*From Weston: Australas Radiol 13:211, 1969.*)

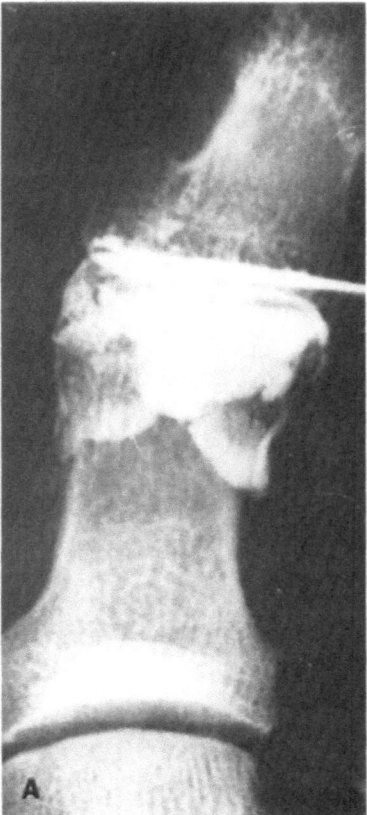
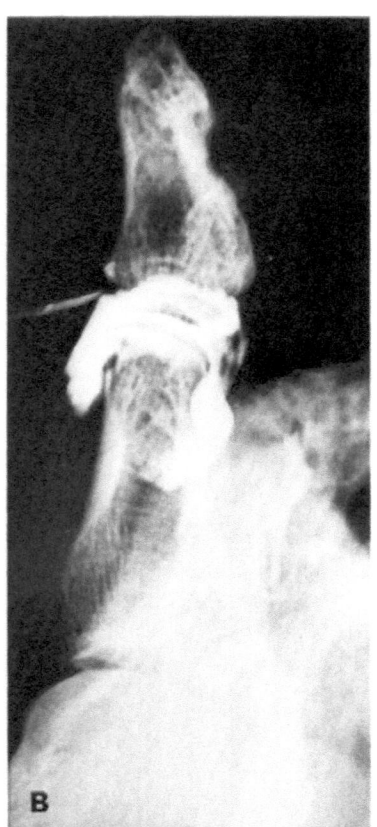

Ganglia are seen in the feet and when adjacent to a joint produce a space-taking lesion which can easily be mistaken for a synovial mass (Fig. 8-13).

Psoriatic arthritis and Reiter's disease both produce a rather distinctive soft tissue change in one or more toes. Diffuse swelling of the whole digit may be present and this is readily appreciated radiologically (Fig. 8-14). The pathologic basis for this change has not been determined; but as both diseases may ultimately produce radiologic evidence of

Fig. 8-12. Posteroanterior (**A**) and oblique (**B**) projections of fractures through the epiphysis of the second and third metatarsals. The widening of the second and third metatarsophalangeal joints is well seen. The fractures are intracapsular. (*From Weston: Australas Radiol 15:367, 1971.*)

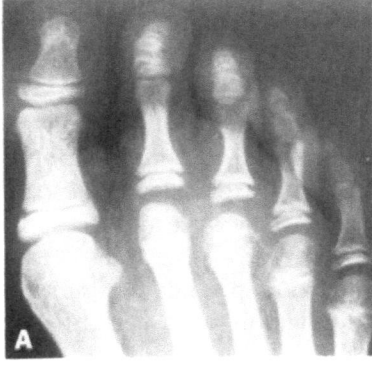
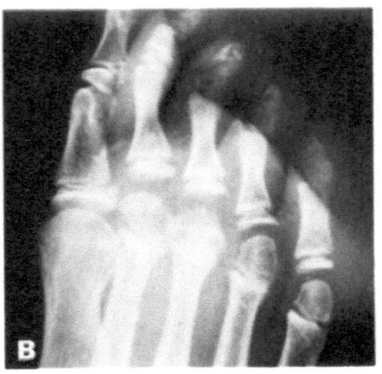

The Tarsus and Foot

Fig. 8-13. A large ganglion forming a soft tissue density adjacent to a metatarsophalangeal joint. **A.** Anteroposterior view. **B.** Lateral view of fore foot.

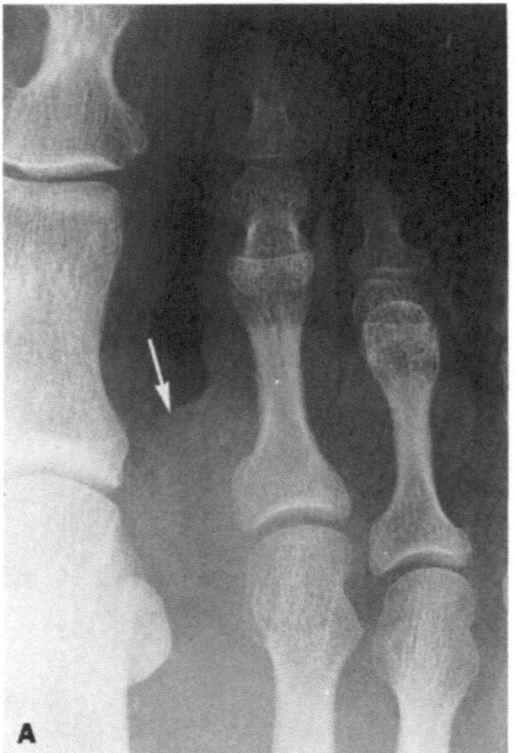

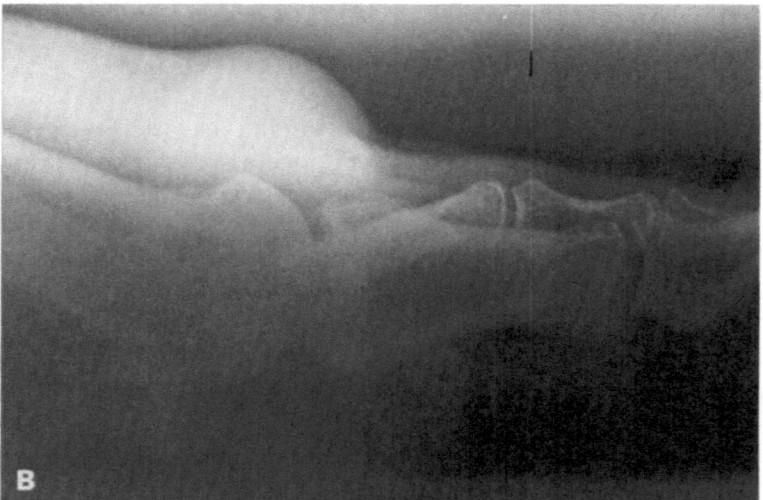

a periostitis it is likely that the diffuse swelling is the result of inflammatory changes along the shafts of the phalanges.

Gout is classically associated with an acute arthritis involving the first metatarsophalangeal joint. In Figure 8-15A the very considerable soft tissue swelling overlying the first metatarsophalangeal joint on the left and the first tarsometatarsal joint on the right is clearly seen. The spread of the inflammatory reaction into the extraarticular tissues is con-

Fig. 8-14. Patient with Reiter's disease with a diffuse, cylindrically swollen second toe of the right foot.

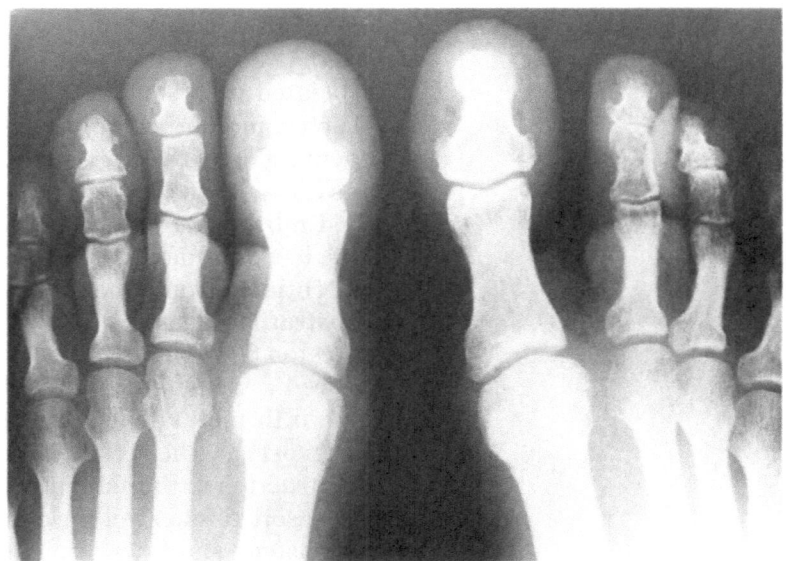

Fig. 8-15. A. Acute gout. There is roentgenographic evidence of an acute inflammatory response involving the right first metatarsophalangeal joint and the left first tarsometatarsal joint. Loss of the fascial–fat interface is shown. **B.** Resolution of the changes seen in **A** with restoration of the fascia–fat interface.

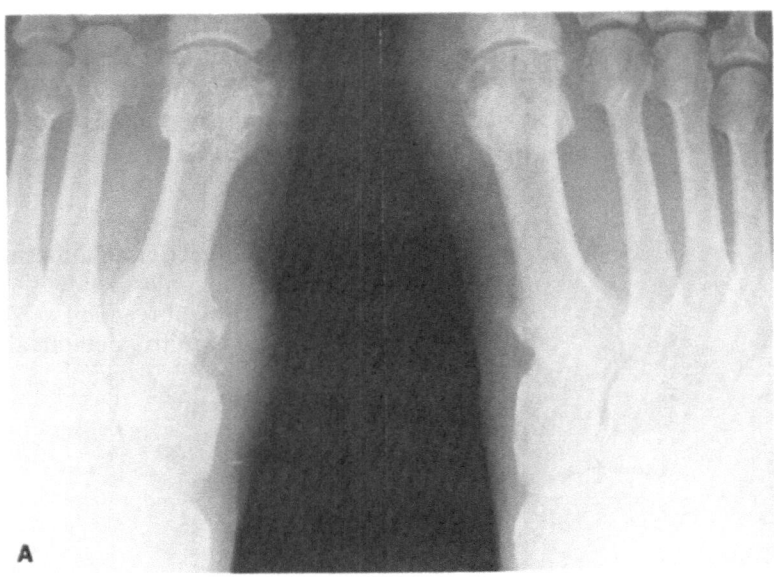

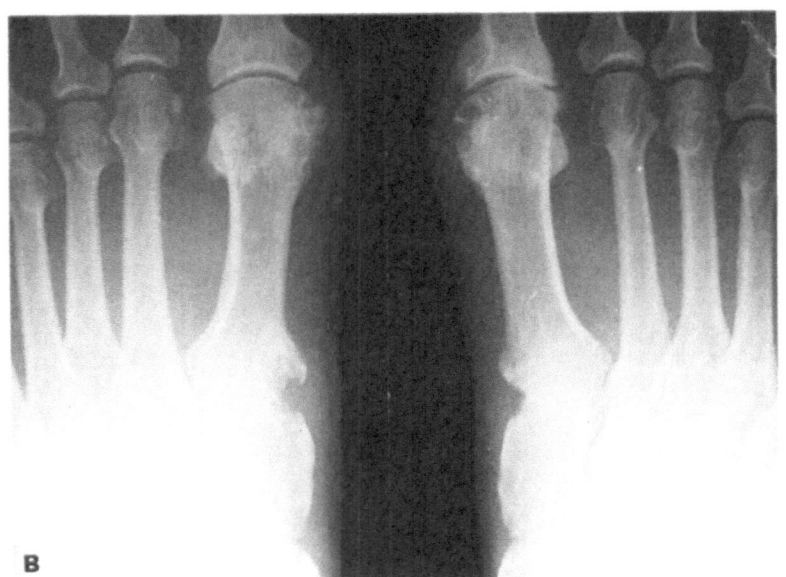

firmed by finding that the boundary between the fascia and fat has been lost. Other forms of erosive arthritis are not associated with such a brisk inflammatory response, nor with such rapid and complete resolution of the reaction as is evident in Figure 8-15B, which shows the appearances after therapy.

Embedded thorns and twigs are most commonly seen in the feet and may induce a reaction which may have to be differentiated from other disease processes (4). Four cases demonstrating various facets of these lesions were described by Weston (7). The first case was due to a box thorn which produced a well-defined area of bone destruction at the base of the fifth metatarsal with well-organized periosteal reaction (Fig. 8-16). The second case was a multilocular area of bone destruction in the cuboid with a thin sclerotic rim. Considerable soft tissue swelling was noted on the radiograph and a persistent sinus was noted clinically. The third case presented with periosteal reaction on the midshaft of the fibula with an underlying translucent oval zone of bone destruction, with associated edema at the site of the sinus. A piece of wood was found in contact with the fibula. The fourth case presented as a mass lesion in quadriceps which was consid-

Fig. 8-16. Reaction to a thorn. Bone destruction associated with a periosteal reaction at the base of the fifth metatarsal. *(From Weston: Br J Radiol 36:323, 1963.)*

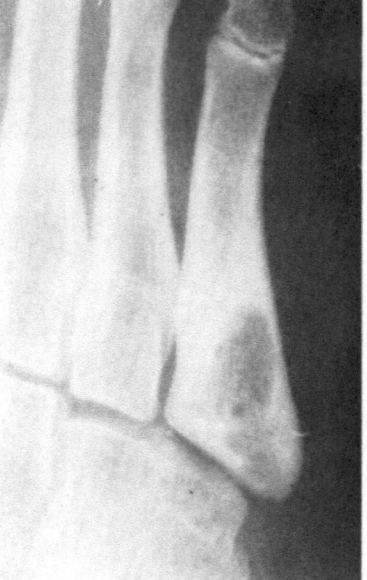

Fig. 8-17. Synovial mass lesion about a metatarsophalangeal joint in patient with rheumatoid arthritis. The mass is irregularly spindle-shaped.

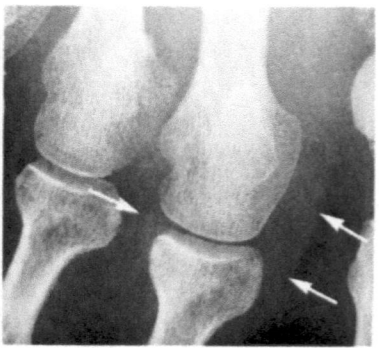

Soft Tissues of the Extremities

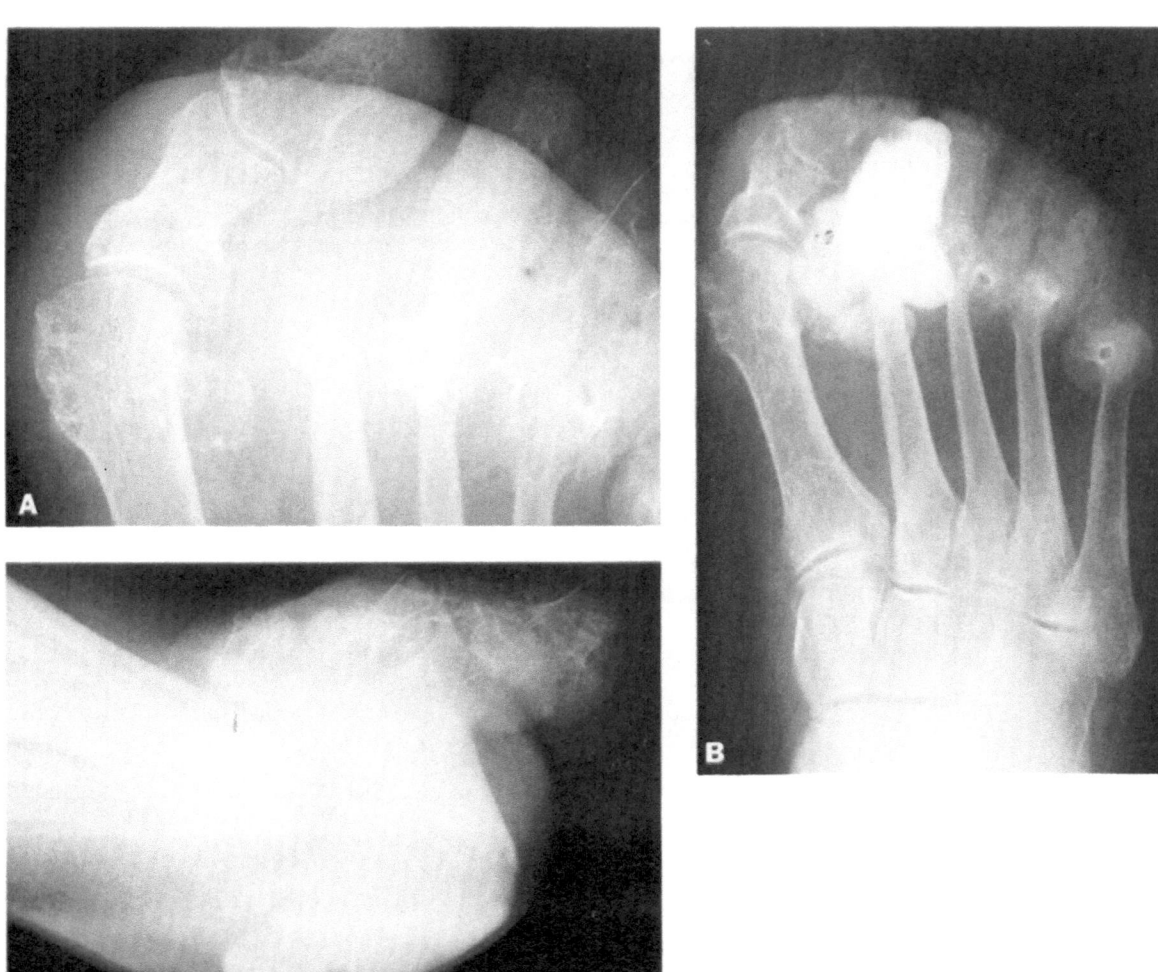

Fig. 8-18. A. A soft tissue mass arising from the second metatarsophalangeal joint due to rheumatoid arthritis. **B.** An arthrogram of the joint shown in **A**. Anteroposterior view. **C.** Lateral view of **B**.

ered as a sarcoma on clinical grounds. No tumor circulation was found on arteriography and marked edema was noted at the fascia–fat interface. A twig from the kowhai tree (Sophora) was found in the necrotic center of this granuloma in the quadriceps.

Rheumatoid Disease

When rheumatoid arthritis involves the metatarsophalangeal and interphalangeal joints the synovial reaction produces

Fig. 8-19. A. Anteroposterior view of an adventitous cyst arising under subluxed metatarsal heads outlined by contrast medium. Rheumatoid disease. **B.** Lateral view of **A**. (*From Palmer: Australas Radiol 14:418, 1970.*)

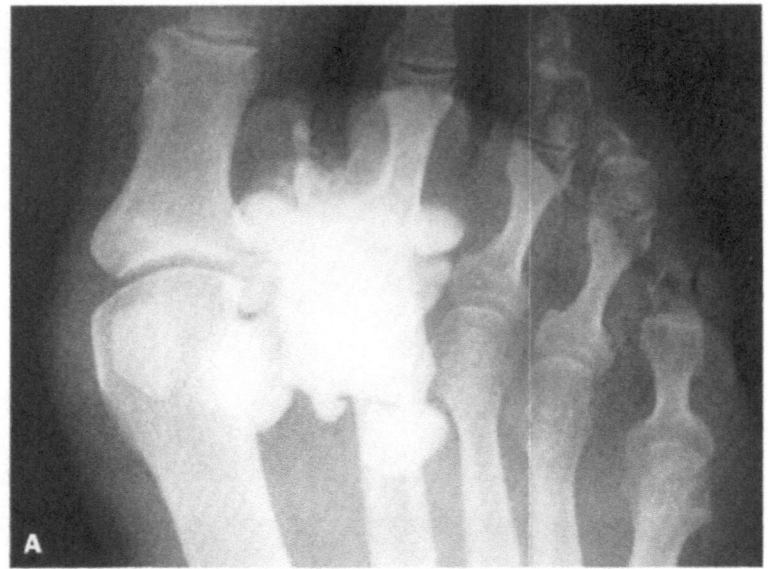

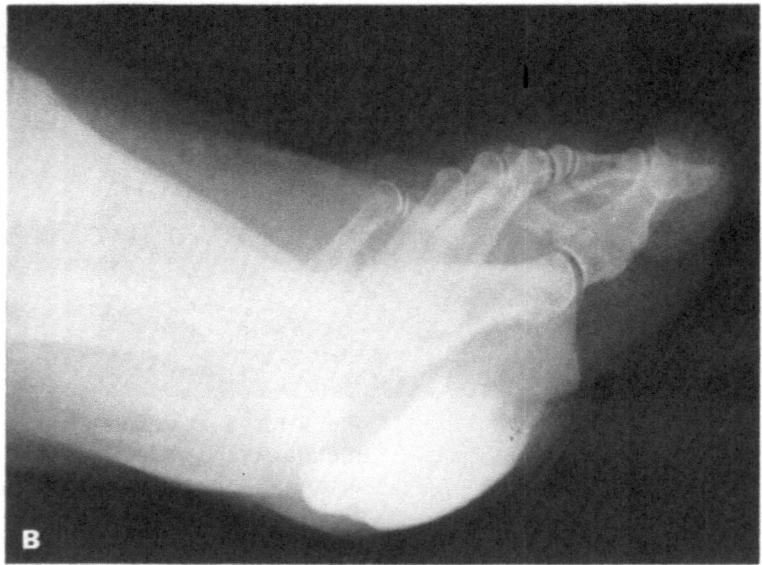

distension of the capsule and the normal box shape (8) becomes replaced by a spindle-shaped mass. This mass can have quite a marked shoulder at the base of the proximal phalanx and can be of sufficient bulk to separate the metatarsal heads (Fig. 8-17). Sacculation of the capsule of a metatarsophalangeal joint can occur producing bizarre appearances (Fig. 8-18A–C). Adventitious bursae may develop under metatarsal heads which have subluxed into the sole. The extent of one such bursa is shown in Fig. 8-19.

Soft Tissues of the Extremities

References

1. Beetham WP, Polley HF, Slocomb CH, et al: Physical Examination of the Joints. Philadelphia, Saunders, 1965, pp 173–174
2. Hansson LJ: Arthrographic studies on ankle joint. Acta Radiol (Stockh) 22:281, 1941
3. Lewis RW: Roentgenographic soft tissue study in an orthopaedic hospital. Am J Roentgenol 48:634, 1942
4. Maylahn DJ: Thorn-induced "tumors" of bone. J Bone Joint Surg [Am] 34:386, 1952
4a. Vainio R: The rheumatoid foot. A clinical study with pathologic and radiologic comments. Ann Chir Gynaecol Fenn (Suppl) 1:16, 1956
5. Weston WJ: Traumatic effusions of the ankle joint and posterior subtaloid joints. Br J Radiol 31:445, 1958
6. Weston WJ: Tendinitis calcarea on the dorsum of the foot. Br J Radiol 32:495, 1959
7. Weston WJ: Thorn and twig-induced pseudotumours of bone and soft tissues. Br J Radiol 36:323, 1963
8. Weston WJ: The normal arthrograms of the metacarpophalangeal, metatarso-phalangeal, and interphalangeal joints. Australas Radiol 13:211, 1969
9. Weston WJ: Positive contrast arthrography of the normal midtarsal joints. Australas Radiol 13:365, 1969
10. Weston WJ: Joint space widening with intracapsular fractures in joints of the fingers and toes of children. Australas Radiol 15:367, 1971
11. Weston WJ: Peroneal tendinitis calcarea. Br J Radiol 32:134, 1959
12. Weston WJ, Antilla P: Synovial lesions of the midtarsal and posterior subtaloid joints in rheumatoid arthritis. Australas Radiol 16:84, 1972

Index

Index

Index

124

Index

Wood Jones, F., 68
Wrist, 48–60
    anteroposterior and lateral projections of, 56
    anatomy of, 48
    "ball-catcher's" view of, 51
    deep fascia in relation to ulnar styloid process
        in, 50
    edema in, 53
    fascia–fat interface in, 48
    fascia–fat plane in, 57–58
    flexor tendons of, 52–53
    full flexion of, 52
    ganglion formation in, 55–57
    hyperextension of, 52
    rheumatoid diseases and, 57–60
    rheumatoid arthritis of, 58
    soft tissue changes of, 53–57
    soft tissue swelling at, 58
    synovial sheaths of flexor tendons of, 52–53
    tendon sheath thickening in, 54
    tendon sheath tumors of, 57

X

Xeroradiography, 3–17
    edge effect in, 3
    resolving power of, 3

Index